The
JACK
DORSEY
Way

**Greater Health, More Energy, A Longer Life:
What the Founder of Twitter Has Discovered,
and How It Can Work For You**

Brad Munson

PERMUTED
PRESS

A PERMUTED PRESS BOOK

ISBN: 978-1-68261-905-6
ISBN (eBook): 978-1-68261-906-3

The Jack Dorsey Way:
Greater Health, More Energy, A Longer Life: What the Founder of
Twitter Has Discovered, And How It Can Work For You

Cover art by Cody Corcoran

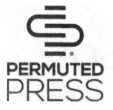

Permuted Press, LLC
New York • Nashville
permutedpress.com

CONTENTS

INTRODUCING THE
JACK DORSEY WAY

Jack Dorsey—billionaire, innovator, disruptor,
college dropout—is the definition of the "self-made
man." But the thing is: He *remakes* himself almost
every day. And maybe you can do the same....

D orsey's amazing transformation into one of the richest
people in America, due to his growing reputation as an
innovator and disruptor, is common knowledge. You
can see him featured on the *Today Show* or *People* magazine;
you can Google his name and get his basic bio in a sentence: A
medium-town boy from St. Louis, a part-time fashion model in
his youth, he started writing code for computers when he was in
middle school; some of the vehicle-dispatching applications he
built way back then are still in use by taxi companies today. He
attended college—first the University of Missouri—Rolla, then
New York University—but he dropped out in 1999, just a few
months before his formal graduation. Soon he was in California
and pitching new ideas, forming new companies, and moving

upward with startling speed. That little idea he had in his last few months at NYU—a short-message "instant messenger" service that could put virtually anyone in touch with anyone else—was already beginning to take shape. The first prototype of Twitter, developed by Dorsey and a contractor named Florian Weber, was used as an internal service for a company called Odeo in 2005; and the first full version premiered on July 15, 2006. The rest is quite literally history. Today, "Twitter" is a household word, like "Kleenex," and the effects it has had in its short life have been truly amazing.

What Jack Dorsey has done in the twenty-plus years since his application arrived has changed the world. Twitter and all its imitators have affected everything from love and marriage to presidential politics. Social media has brought people together and helped them accomplish extraordinary things. In the same way, it has also driven us apart. And Dorsey has been at the center of it since the very beginning, as very few others have been.

Today, he is the (second time around) CEO of Twitter and its e-commerce partner, Square. He runs the company, travels the world, and still regularly reports on his continuing dedication to leading a surprising, productive, high-quality life on a day-to-day basis through his own social media accounts and journals. And he does it all in public, where we can all see it... and where many feel free to criticize and comment.

Jack Dorsey isn't the only billion-dollar entrepreneur with a unique and very public set of health and wellness practices. Everyone from *Shark Tank* star Mark Cuban, to ninety-five-year-old Charlie Munger, to Tony Robbins has something to say about staying healthy and living a long time; but Dorsey is a little different. All along the way, Jack Dorsey has proven himself to be something more than simply another "billionaire of the month" eccentric. True, he has a tendency to use a lot of jargon—words like being "performant" and "clear" to achieve his remarkable level of energy and accomplishment. But what's far more important is that he is *constantly evolving*. Dorsey has never settled on a single "thing," a single strategy or point of view. He's always trying new things, replacing old tactics with new ones, and his enthusiasm for this forward-facing (and sometime under-critical) approach never flags.

One thing that has remained consistent throughout Dorsey's bodyhacking adventures is a singular, unwavering commitment to *mindfulness*. Since long ago, since the days before anyone knew who Jack Dorsey was, and when "twitter" was still just a sound effect for songbirds, he has cared deeply about *paying attention* to every decision he makes: what he eats, how and when and how much he moves, how he experiences the world and how he fits into it. And he has regularly documented, written about, talked about, and shared all of it That's what makes it special…and useful.

Now, at least for a little while, we're going to join Jack Dorsey on his journey. We're going to look at a number of elements of his lifestyle that he swears by, recommends, and repeats in public often. But we're not simply going to accept that everything he says or has tried is right for everyone, or even for him—otherwise we'd all eating nothing but purple foods.

Instead, we're going to use Jack Dorsey's observations and practices as a series of springboards—of ideas that we'll explore from the ground up, and work with, to see just how much they can apply to your own particular situation, your own unique needs and goals. The plan is for you to learn a great deal about yourself and your potential along the way, and to leave the experience with some great new ideas and inspiration on how *you* can change your life—and the world around you—just like Jack Dorsey has and continues to do.

Let's get started....

HOW TO USE THIS BOOK

t would be easy just to cobble together a bunch of articles or blogs about each of the elements in Jack Dorsey's Way. But that wouldn't serve you well...and frankly, it wouldn't be safe. There's nothing overtly dangerous or contraindicated about the things that Dorsey does...but they also offer us lessons in *practicality* and *moderation.*

Many of the habits that are part of Dorsey's everyday life are relatively easy to achieve—walking to work a couple of days a week, monitoring your sleep, meditation. Others are a little more exotic and can lead to great expense. We'll try to deal with those issues as we go along. But as you browse through this book, and dig into the parts that matter the most to you individually, keep a few things in mind:

One Size Does Not Fit All

There's a very popular term among doctors and health professionals these days. Everybody's talking about the *microbiome,* often—confusingly—abbreviated to the *biome.*

Strictly speaking, the microbiome is the collection of microbes—bacteria, fungi, viruses, protozoa, and more—that live inside you, infiltrating and surrounding your cells. In fact, we have about ten times more microbes in our body—all those constituent parts of the microbiome—than we actually have cells. And rather like fingerprints, your microbiome is absolutely unique. What diseases you've had and been exposed to, your genetic makeup, your eating patterns, the place you live, the actual structure of your cells, muscles, and brain tissue all affect that personal microscopic "fingerprint." It's basically a very impressive way to say that *every one of us is different,* right down to the subcellular level.

In practical terms, we see that expressed every day in things like allergies and personal immunities. Externally, any dozen people may *look* identical; they may even be genetically related, or live in the same apartment complex, or work in the same building. But each of them will respond to the foods they eat; the medications they take; the stress levels they experience; even their exposure to light, color, sound, and temperature in entirely different ways.

That's why one of the few general statements you can trust is, "Don't Trust General Statements." What works perfectly for Person A—even someone of the same gender, ethnicity, age, weight, and even family—may not work for you at all. You may respond to that bit of exercise advice, that food, or that "habit" in an entirely different way.

We all long for simple, straightforward answers—for the magic pill, the "silver bullet." But if modern medical science has learned anything, it has learned—and doctors will grudgingly but almost universally admit this—that everyone is different; that nothing works for everyone.

So be careful in treating anything on Jack Dorsey's list as absolute or automatically "right" for you. Realize that you will be tailoring what you learn here and elsewhere to your own specific needs and requirements—to your own *microbiome*— from the very beginning. And we will talk a bit in a minute about how you can go about that "tailoring" process in a relatively painless way.

"Too Much of a Good Thing" Is Too True

Clichés can be awfully boring, and just because something has been said a million times, doesn't make it true...but here is one boring old cliché that actually proves out: "*Moderation is a virtue.*"

On its surface, some of Jack Dorsey's approaches are rather extreme: one meal a day, intermittent fasting, even the physical extremes of ice baths. Many of these tactics may work very well for you...but keep in mind that there is a limit to what works and how "scalable" it is. For instance, there is a great deal of evidence to indicate that seven-minute high-intensity workouts are a good thing; they can produce and maintain muscle mass very well and can improve your cardiovascular system's efficiency over the short and long term. But that doesn't mean a *fourteen-minute* high-intensity workout will improve your physical form *twice* as well as a seven-minute strategy. In fact, if you ramp up that tactic too much, you can actually do yourself more damage than good.

The same applies to intermittent fasting. As we'll see, there is growing evidence, and even some common sense, that indicates it can be an important and effective tool in mindful eating, weight loss, and healthy weight maintenance. Taken to the extreme—beyond the boundaries of moderation—extreme fasting can become obsessive and result in an eating disorder that does not serve you, your body, or the people you care about.

As you consider integrating some or all of the Jack Dorsey Way into your everyday life-habits, keep *moderation* in mind. Remember the words of Norwegian author and intellectual Jostein Gaarder, who said, "Health is the natural condition. When sickness occurs, it is a sign that Nature has gone off course because of a physical or mental imbalance. The road to health for everyone is through moderation, harmony, and a 'sound mind in a sound body'."

(And of course, the occasional splurge or "vacation" can do wonders for you as well. As you're remembering Gaarder, remember American philosopher Ralph Waldo Emerson as well: "Moderation in all things, especially moderation.")

The More We Learn, The More We Change

If you've picked up this book, if you've gotten this far, you're obviously looking to change your life for the better. That's a good thing, but it's not necessarily an *easy* thing. Profound change takes time, self-discipline, and—worst of all—*patience.*

Keep in mind that Jack Dorsey does the things we cover in this book *every day,* or at the very least, a few times a week. He's done them, in some cases, for years, and the results have not necessarily been rapid or immediately noticeable.

So what he practices, and what we discuss here, isn't presented as a set of short-term quick fixes. This isn't *Build a Sexier Body in 28 Days*. This is an attempt to change the way you live *permanently*. It is much more a matter of *evolution* than sudden, drastic *transformation*.

Additionally, remember that what works for you today won't necessarily be working for you nearly as well—or at all—a month from now or a year from now. At an intellectual and spiritual level, we are constantly evolving and ascending—or at least we hope we are—and what seems like a "perfect" bit of advice or a life-strategy for us at age eighteen may seem entirely inappropriate for us at age eighty. By the same token, our bodies are constantly adjusting and re-adjusting to changes in diet, routine, and levels of physical activity; and the effects of those changes on your body and mind can change over time as well.

Take, for example, the recently identified and confirmed concept of "plateauing" in weight loss. For most people, it is relatively simple to adopt one of many "diets" or exercise plans and lose five to seven percent of your body weight no matter what that body weight might be. But it is equally likely, overwhelmingly likely, that once you have achieved that percentage of weight loss, your body will begin to generate a whole host of hormones—which will actually change your brain chemistry!— to convince you that you're losing *too much weight too quickly*. You will suddenly feel hungrier than you ever have before; you will find it harder and harder to feel full (what nutritionists call "satiety"). And you will find it increasingly difficult to stop thinking about food, especially your favorite foods. This is known as "perseverance" by the experts, complete with its own odd pronunciation.

The result: you will stop losing weight so quickly. You will *plateau*. This isn't simply a matter of "willpower" or some great psychological flaw. This is biochemistry. Your body has been triggered by your sudden weight loss. Its deep programming thinks something is wrong, that there is a threat to your survival because you have decreased your normal food intake and increased your physical activity. So your body is changing itself to protect you. It is *learning*…and in this case, unfortunately, it is learning the wrong lesson.

The point is: We, as individuals, are in a constant state of change, and much of that change is beyond our control. This means that any decision we make about how to take care of ourselves is a *temporary* decision, whether we want it to be or not, and those choices need to be reassessed on a regular basis. Jack Dorsey himself knows this; that is why he continues to try new things and modify old strategies and tactics, because way down deep as well as right up to: *things change*. And the more we learn, the more we change, at a "brain" level and at a "body" level.

At the end of this book, you'll find a list of resources that were current on the date of publication. They are provided to you precisely because we know that things *do* change—we learn new things and try new things all the time.

TMAC: A Tried and True Strategy for Change

Trying new things can be hard. Making decisions about what to try and when to say "pass" can be equally hard. And the toughest challenge of all can be sticking with the decisions you make.

There is one time-tested tool that can help you in this process. It's generally known by the acronym of TMAC, and as you're digging deeper into The Jack Dorsey Way, it's a process you may find very helpful.

TMAC stands for:

- Test
- Measure
- Assess
- Commit

Let's discuss each of those elements very quickly.

Test. There's no need to jump head-first into any one of the approaches that Jack Dorsey uses. Read up on one of them first, and if it appeals to you, *test it*. Try to put together a version that works for you *temporarily*, and attempt it for a significant period of time...but not yet forever.

Try to set it up as a classic experiment from science class. Ask yourself, "What questions do I want answered?" "How will I know when it's answered?" "How will I structure my experiment?" (More on that in a minute.)

This may seem like a lot of work at first, but it's worth it. Treating your life-change as a test will lower your expectations in a good way; if you look at it as a *test* at first, rather than as a permanent, abrupt, and fundamentally risky life-change, then you won't feel like a "failure" if this particular tactic doesn't "take" with you. *Testing* is a learning process that focuses on the information you gain from the test, not on the often-debilitating concept of *success* or *failure*.

For instance: you may want to *test* the idea of walking to work (or to the market or in the woods) two times a week for, say, three months. Anything less than three to six months probably isn't long enough to let the "new" feel of the strategy wear off, and for a realistic level of self-awareness to sink in. It's also unlikely that any positive results from any of the Jack Dorsey Way strategies will yield noticeable, attributable results in anything less than that time period.

If after a month you find that you just can't manage to make time for that twice-weekly walk, no matter how hard you try, then you've learned something. If you still want to pursue that goal, you now know that you'll have to change something about the way you're approaching it—the time of day, the days you've chosen, the destination, and so on. You haven't *failed* at anything. You've *learned,* and that's far better for you both psychologically and in terms of real results.

Measure. When you decide on your test, decide on exactly what you're going to measure as an indicator of your goal. Do you want to lose, say, ten pounds in two months? Do you want to lower your heart rate by twenty percent? Do you want to sleep for at least two hours more a night? The measurement—in current, common parlance, the *metric*—needs to be something specific and quantifiable; a *number,* not just a feeling. You can't measure "feeling better" or "feeling happier," but you *can* measure "pounds of ice cream consumed in a week," or "miles walked in a month." So choose your metric and keep a record.

That's the other thing: *Keep a record.* Don't rely on your faulty human memory. Use a bit of wearable tech or a good old-fashioned journal to measure your progress on a regular basis—and no fudging, even if the measurements are different than what you'd hoped. This kind of record keeping will not only give you hard evidence for the next step, but as you improve—and you will!—it will give you a solid basis for celebration and further motivation. You will see your "numbers" improving, and that is a huge psychological booster.

Assess. Now, take the measurements you've made during your test and closely examine them—*assess* them. Try to separate them from your personal sense of accomplishment or lack thereof; try your very best to leave your ego and expectation at the door and just look at the facts: your quantifiable goals and your numbers.

This can be the hardest part of the entire TMAC process. You began this entire adventure because you wanted to change for the better—you wanted to reach your goal. And it can be very difficult when the numbers aren't what you want, when things aren't changing the way you want them to or as quickly as you had hoped. Still, be brutally honest.

Look at the numbers and the goal, not at your feelings. And *assess* whether this approach to your health and wellness is something to commit to, or alter and try again, or to pass by and move on.

There are no wrong answers here. The only mistake you can make is to not decide.

Then, finally, if the assessment calls for it, it's time to…

Commit. As we've said before, the ultimate goal here is *long-term evolution,* not short-term Band-Aids. So if one or more of these strategies or tactics of the Jack Dorsey Way appeals to you, and you've properly tested it, measured it, and assessed the results, the next and final question to ask yourself is, *Can I do this for the rest of my life?*…or at the very least *for the foreseeable future?* (A loaded term, yes, but you get the idea.)

Maybe because of your excitement or interest, you were able to achieve the desired results during your test period. But be honest with yourself: Is this something (like eating one meal a day or taking ice baths) that you want to do for years to come?

It's a matter of both practicality and preference. Does your neighborhood or your geographical location make twice-weekly walking to work viable year-round? Do you dread one more dip in the ice bath, or have you come to actually enjoy it and look forward to it?

Here again: Be brutally honest. A lukewarm concession, even a private one made only to yourself, along the lines of, "Well, I'll try it for a few weeks and see how it goes," probably isn't adequate at this point. You've already been through that; you've tested for months already; you know what the effects are and you know, deep down, how you feel about this particular process. So decide. For real, forever (or at least the foreseeable forever.) And only *then* should you make this commitment, and carry on.

TMAC breaks down these big life decisions into manageable parts—steps you can endure without permanent damage to your ego or your body. So consider using this tool as you look at the various elements in the Jack Dorsey Way.

And all that being said…let's start the journey!

The Dorsey Way: A Checklist

- **Meditating Twice a Day**
- **Walking to Work**
- **Seven-Minute High-Intensity Interval Training (HIIT)**
- **Saunas and Ice Baths (Starting the day with an ice-cold bath, too)**
- **A Standing Desk**
- **Near-Infrared Rays**
- **Eating One Meal per Day and Weekend Fasts**
- **Daily Vitamin and Mineral Supplements**
- **Monitoring Sleep**
- **Journaling**

MEDITATION

**The Jack Dorsey Way: Dorsey tries to
meditate for an hour every morning, right after waking up
shortly after 6:00 a.m., and for an additional hour every night.**

Throughout his years of lifestyle "experimentation," Jack Dorsey has consistently included *meditation* in his day-to-day practices. He has often said that it has had the single greatest impact on him in terms of mental health, over and above any of the other practices he's undertaken in his ongoing attempt to improve his life. In fact, he has practiced daily meditation in one form or another for more than twenty years—half his life—and in recent years has become more dedicated to it than ever before. What began as mere five-minute breaks in the routine has become a major commitment for Dorsey, as he has become focused on the specific meditation practice calls *Vipassanā* (which we'll discuss in greater detail a bit later). On a recent podcast, Dorsey has said, "a lot of my routine today is all due to what felt like just had to be done in order to, not only survive but to make sure that I continue to be performing and continue to be clear."

What Is Meditation?

Many of the other elements in Jack Dorsey's regimen are self-explanatory: daily walks, ice baths, fasts, and the rest. But *meditation* is unique in its wide use and equally widespread misunderstanding, often by those who use it.

What is meditation, exactly?

At its center, meditation is a *practice,* a set of self-directed, intentional habits or mental behaviors intended to create a particular state of mind. Overall, the goal of meditation, in all its many forms, is to create an ongoing calm and insightful state of mind, to achieve and maintain a state of mental and spiritual tranquility and balance that will have a positive effect on your physical as well as your psycho-spiritual well-being, forging and reinforcing an expanding and healthy connection between body and mind.

In other words, meditation is a process of *training your mind,* and though the specific tools and strategies differ from discipline to discipline and teacher to teacher, it is a process that is accessible to nearly everyone, at any age, at any level of income, education, or ability.

There are many types of meditation—some very old, some relatively new—but they all share a few characteristics:

- **A singular focus,** on a particular and carefully chosen word or phrase, or an object, or on breathing itself.

- **A consistent, comfortable physical posture,** whether that means lying down, sitting, or even walking. Stressful change in body position or use is counter-productive.
- **Lack of distraction.** Though the location may differ from individual to individual, or even from day to day, the "space" chosen for meditation should be quiet, uncluttered, and free of visual and aural distraction.
- **A relaxed and open attitude,** one that accepts the inevitable distractions, from noise to errant thoughts to upwelling anxieties, and lets them pass through the mind rather than disturb the state of being. It is quite literally the process of letting yourself "go with the flow."

Though meditation has existed in many forms for a very long time, it has become a "mainstream" practice in the U.S. only in recent years. A report from the National Health Interview Service found that the use of meditation among adults in the United States *tripled* from 2012 to 2017, and it's been growing ever since. It's probably safe to say that one out of five Americans now practice some form of meditation on a regular basis—more than ever before. And the use of meditation by children under the age of seventeen has grown even more, and more quickly.

This may be in part because so many famous and successful people now talk openly about their use of meditation. Oprah Winfrey, Hugh Jackman, Richard Branson, Paul McCartney, Angelina Jolie, Michael Jordan, Misty May-Treanor, Derek Jeter, Rupert Murdoch, Russell Simmons, Arnold Schwarzenegger,

Eva Mendes, and Arianna Huffington all practice meditation. Check our "Resources" section for an ever-growing list.

What Can Meditation Do For You?

If you study meditation in any form, even a little, you will find an awesome array of claims about its benefits, from extending your life to curing cancer. While many of these claims remain unproven (and in some cases unprovable), the remarkable fact is that a wide range of scientific studies have shown that a consistent practice of meditation can, in fact, have powerful positive effects on the quality of life, both mentally and physically.

Among the many proven benefits:

Stress reduction. More than one study has found that meditation, or *mindfulness* (a word you will see often in your reading and research), can measurably reduce the symptoms of stress. In fact, meditation may actually physically reduce the density of brain tissue that is associated with anxiety.

The biochemical origins of stress are complex to say the least, but one well-known culprit is a hormone called *cortisol*, which creates—among other things—a family of chemicals called *cytokines* that promote inflammation, disrupt sleep, promote depression and anxiety, and interfere with clear thinking. More than one carefully designed and controlled study has shown that meditation can measurably reduce this inflammatory response, especially among those with the highest levels of stress.

Reduction in blood pressure. This particular positive effect of meditation is probably the most studied and solid claim of all. A great many studies show that meditative practices, like concentrating on a "silent mantra," can reduce blood pressure by significant amounts. It's generally felt that meditation relaxes the nerve signals that coordinate heart function, reduces the tension in blood vessels, and avoids the triggering of the "fight-or-flight" response that occurs in stressful situations. So the positive effect not only improves the meditator's numbers when it comes to blood pressure, also known as *hypertension*, but reduces the strain on the entirely cardiovascular system, helping to reduce the risk of heart disease.

The reduction of physical pain. Chronic pain, even in "healthy" people, is a huge problem in the modern world, and controlling it is a major challenge. Obviously medications can help, but over the years—and again, currently, with the opioid crisis—we're seeing the dangers of relying too heavily of drugs alone to help control pain. That's why so much attention has been paid to the use of meditation in pain reduction, and a wide range of studies have shown—amazingly enough—that meditation may actually work better than morphine itself, the mother of all pain drugs. Various studies show a measurable reduction in physical pain related to a wide range of conditions, including irritable bowel syndrome, ulcerative colitis, fibromyalgia, multiple sclerosis, and many others.

Relief of anxiety and depression. The effects of consistent meditative practice are closely related to the issues of stress, but there have also been a number of studies that specifically address meditation's effect on depression and again have found strong clinical evidence of its beneficial properties. It has also been proven to reduce symptoms of anxiety disorders, including phobias, social anxiety, paranoid thoughts, obsessive-compulsive behaviors, and panic attacks. Even more subtle challenges, like job-related anxiety, can be reduced; and many studies have shown that the positive effects are not only immediate, but long-term.

Help with insomnia and other sleep disorders. It is sad but true: Nearly half the population of the United States, and by extension the Western World at large, will struggle with insomnia at some point in their lives. And here again, meditation has proven to help people fall asleep sooner, stay asleep longer, and achieve beneficial and healing REM sleep more easily and for longer periods of time compared to those who do not meditate. Again, stress-related biochemistry is a factor, but the practice of meditation itself also comes into play. After all, practicing meditation means *controlling* or *redirecting your thoughts*, and if you can actively participate in the process of relaxing, releasing tension, and placing yourself in a peaceful state of mind, you will certainly help yourself fall asleep and sleep better.

Help with the struggle against addiction. Though this claim remains controversial and needs additional research, it is fairly well-established that meditation can help people overcome addictive behavior. One study that focused on the *Vipassanā* meditative practice—the school that Jack Dorsey is currently involved with—showed it to be very effective in helping people overcome alcohol and drug-related addictions. Other forms of meditation, examined in other studies, have proven effective as well. The mindfulness that is part of meditation may be part of the explanation; in meditation, you are able not only to increase your self-control, but you become more aware of the factors in your personal environment that trigger specific behaviors—addictive behaviors included. Meditation can help redirect one's attention, leading to better control of impulses and personal understanding. And this can apply to a wide range of addictive behaviors that go beyond drugs and alcohol into eating disorders, including binge eating.

An improvement of the immune system. *Inflammation* is a widely used buzzword in traditional and alternative medicine these days, but it is a real and measurable presence in the human body, and it does its greatest damage to the immune system, your bulwark against infection and chronic disease. Recent randomized trials from major institutions indicate that meditation has a consistently positive influence on the production of cytokines and other chemicals that promote inflammation, so the reduction of those chemicals through meditation has already been shown to help your body fight off disease and increase the speed and power of healing.

...and though it is far more difficult to scientifically measure, the overwhelming anecdotal evidence is that meditation improves the *quality* of your life as well. Millions of people who use meditation daily will tell you it increases your sense of well-being, gives you access to greater energy, makes you more creative, even improves your memory. Certainly Jack Dorsey ascribes to these beliefs when he says it is a key element to feeling more "performative" and "clear" every day.

Why is meditation so effective? It may be, in part, because pain is partly a matter of *perception*, which is highly affected by your state of mind, and meditation can alter that state of mind for the better. One study used Magnetic Resonance Imaging, or MRI, to observe brain activity in subjects who were experiencing a painful stimulus. The test group in the study had been given four days of mindfulness meditation training, while the control group had not...and the subjects who received training in meditative techniques showed increased brain activity in the centers that control pain, as well as reportedly less sensitivity to pain itself. These outcomes have been replicated and echoed in other studies looking at chronic and intermittent pain and seem to be especially effective for the elderly and even with those in the final stages of life.

Generally speaking, scientific studies show us that meditation is considered safe for healthy people. However, if your chosen meditative practice includes movement, you should take any existing physical limitations into account before you begin, and a visit to your primary care provider would be a good thing. The same applies to people who are already coping with psychiatric issues relating to anxiety and depression. It's quite unlikely that your mental health caregiver will advise against such a widely used and respected practice as meditation, but checking first is still worthwhile. You'll probably find that consultation results in great encouragement and even guidance. And of course, meditation is meant to be included in a wide, integrative self-care program. It shouldn't be used to replace conventional care, or as an excuse to delay seeing a healthcare provider about a serious or ongoing medical or mental health issue. Use it as part of the solution, not a cure-all.

Where Did Meditation Originate, and How Did It Come to America?

Meditation, like prayer, is one of the oldest spiritual and psychological disciplines in human history. In the West, its origins can be seen in writings that predate the ancient Greeks. It was Thales, who lived more than six hundred years before Christ, who first memorialized the basic concept of "a sound mind in a sound body"—the essence of the "mind/body connection." A thousand years later, the same notion was encapsulated by the sixteenth century French philosopher Michel de Montaigne, when he said, "The greatest thing in the world is to know how to belong to oneself." Meanwhile, the word "meditation" itself derives directly from the Latin word that means "to ponder."

Some of the oldest written records in the world, originating in Indian culture dating back to fifteen hundred years before Christ, refer to the training of the mind. The Hindu traditions of Vedantism, Buddhist scriptures, and other equally ancient sources reference these disciplines as well. Early forms of meditation are described in Chinese texts; they use terms that will be very familiar to even the most casual student of meditation—terms like "embracing the one," "guarding tranquility," and "embracing simplicity."

No one really knows where meditation "started." It is nearly unique in its presence across so many ancient cultures, under a variety of names. You will find meditative-like practices in Islam, Christianity, and Judaism, as well as in the Eastern philosophies and religions.

The first appearance of meditative principles in Western society can be traced back to the 1700s, when Indian texts like *The Upanishads*—written five hundred to eight hundred years before the birth of Christ—and *The Bhagavad Gita*, a collection of sacred Sanskrit verses from the Hindu epic the *Mahabharata*, circulated widely in the pre-Revolutionary American Colonies. Meditation was explored and discussed by intellectuals and philosophers like Voltaire and Schopenhauer, but it wasn't until the mid-twentieth century that it gained real prominence in North American culture.

Meditation has always been influenced by the culture in which is thrives. Here in the West, with its strong non-secular influences, meditation became far more removed from its religious origins; by the mid-twentieth century, it was being studied extensively using the Western scientific method. Its first widespread appearance came in the 1960s and '70s with the arrival of "Transcendental Meditation," and its embrace by a variety of celebrities and performers; it wasn't until almost the turn of the century that meditation truly entered the mainstream. One author more than any other is responsible for this migration:

Deepak Chopra, whose 1993 book, *Ageless Body, Timeless Mind*, became a bestseller after being endorsed by Oprah Winfrey. Soon thereafter, the highly related concepts of *mindfulness* and *cognitive behavior therapy* further "legitimized" a practice that has been present in societies worldwide for thousands of years. Today, as we said earlier, the number of adults and children from every walk of life who practice meditation in a regular basis is growing, and there is no end in sight.

What Are the Different Kinds of Meditation?

Like any ancient tradition, the practice of meditation has evolved differently in different societies, acquiring various approaches and terminology along the way. There are thousands of books describing different schools of thought. These practices can break down into a few broad categories, each one focusing on specific techniques or strategies that are meant to achieve the common goals of self-awareness, self-understanding, tranquility, and empathy:

- **Mindfulness meditation** focuses on the non-judgmental passage of thoughts through your mind. It often involves focusing on an object or your breath. Originating in Buddhist philosophy, mindfulness meditation is one of the most popular approaches in Western culture.
- **Spiritual meditation** has its roots in Daoism, Hinduism, and even Christianity. It emphases silent

reflection and a deeper connection to your personal version of God. To some, it is the meditative practice that most resembles prayer.

- **Focused meditation** concentrates on the five senses, which can include tools like counting beads, listening to a gong, counting breaths, or even staring at a candle flame. It requires—or develops—great internal discipline.

- **Movement meditation** includes some forms of yoga, but it is in fact richer and deeper than that. Everything from tai chi (also known as qigong) to gardening, or even a tranquil walk in the wilderness, is a form of movement meditation. It encompasses a discipline in which physical movement is an integral part of the meditative practice.

- **Mantra meditation,** very common in Buddhist and Hindu tradition, uses repetitive sounds as a focal point to help the student enter and maintain a meditative state. The classic—almost cliché—notion of *Om* comes from the traditions of mantra meditation.

These various elements commingle and recombine with every teacher, school, and text. As you explore, you will find yourself drawn to a particular set of practices that work best for you—a selection that will almost certainly change as your time practicing meditation, in all its forms, extends through your life.

The Mystery and Effects of Stress

Stress isn't just part of our modern, everyday lives; it's *always* been part of *everyone's* life, back to prehistoric times, and it's actually necessary and beneficial—when used in the right way and in the right quantities. But out-of-control stress can lead to all sorts of negative health issues, from an increase in heart disease, to migraines, to depression. Yet some people seem to deal with it easily, even welcome it, while it does terrible damage to the rest of us.

Why?

Many scientists think the key factor may be *serotonin*, a neurotransmitter that seems to appear less often in people who are prone to depression...and now there may be ways to "map" the creation and use of that and other stress-related brain chemicals.

A study from the University of California San Diego published in the *Journal of Neuroscience* reported on rats that developed the inability to feel pleasure had *more* serotonin-producing neurons in their brains. This may seem to point in the opposite direction, but what it does tell us is that depression is connected to the ability to feel pleasure.

Dr. Nandkishore Prakash, who worked on the study, put the question and answer this way: "Why does stress not lead to symptoms of depression in every stressed individual? We now know that the serotonergic system demonstrates a form of plasticity, hitherto unknown, that is strongly correlated to the behavioral susceptibility of a rodent to stress-induced depression." In simpler English: Some brains are better at recruiting cells for pleasure than others in response to stressful situations, confirming the idea that the brain behaves differently after stress, actually producing different "coping chemicals" in different individuals.

Maybe one day we will be able to identify the molecular marker that makes some people prone to stress-damage and others more resilient to it. But the important lesson to learn so far is that stress-reactions are not entirely psychological—not simply a result

29

of your own history, training, or intent. There is an inevitable and barely understood *physiological* process taking place as well—one we are just beginning to address—which makes stress an even more serious issue.

Ultimately, it *is* all in your head...just not in the way we've always thought.

On *Vipassanā* Meditation

Most recently, Jack Dorsey has concentrated his explorations in meditation on the *Vipassanā* method. As he's said in his own tweets, "Meditation is often thought of as calming, relaxing, and a detox of all the noise in the world. That's not *Vipassanā*. It's extremely painful and demanding physical and mental work. I wasn't expecting any of that my first time last year. Even tougher this year as I went deeper."

The word *Vipassanā* means "meditation involving concentration on the body or its sensations, or the insight which this provides," and it is one of India's oldest and most respected forms of meditation; it has been taught in India for more than two thousand years. One of its key elements is an annual ten-day retreat, where participants learn and practice the basics of the method and experience its results.

As Jack Dorsey himself described in various social media, "during the ten days: no devices, reading, writing, physical exercise, music, intoxicants, meat, talking, or even eye contact with others." Even the economic stress is relieved. "It's free," Dorsey said. "Everything is given to meditators by charity." As one popular *Vipassanā* website, Dhamma.org, explains, "All expenses are met by donations from people who, having completed a course and experienced the benefits of *Vipassanā*, wish to give others the opportunity to benefit from it also."

Courses in *Vipassanā* are available in Meditation Centers across the country and around the world. You'll find an alphabetical list of worldwide course locations in our Resources section at the end of this book.

What to Read, How to Find a Teacher

In this one way, if no other, learning meditation is like horse-back riding. It is *possible* to learn it from reading a book without ever actually going near a horse or having a teacher, but it is so much more enlightening, efficient, and rewarding to find the right person, the right class, the right environment, so you can learn what you *really* need to get started.

So how *do* you begin?

First, decide on what style appeals to you most. Attend a few classes, read a bit. Find a local "new age" bookstore or visit one of the many online sites and do some browsing. It doesn't have to be a permanent commitment—in fact, it *shouldn't* be, this early in your journey—but start with some decisions that "speak" to you.

As Meditation advisor Lodro Rinzler says, "A good teacher will simply embody the teachings. They will be present, kind, and open-hearted with you. They will have done the 'work,' so-to-speak, so you are less tempted to ask about the benefits of meditation because you see it in their very being and are inspired. If you can find a teacher like that, cherish this spiritual friend, as they are quite rare."

Writer Stephan Bodian says you may have to confront some of your own preconceptions about a "spiritual teacher" as you find your own. "Perhaps you envision a cloistered monastic dressed in earth-colored robes who gives you spiritual counsel in hushed tones and then returns to his cell to continue his practice. Or maybe you think of a joyful, expansive being who lives in the world and radiates love and light wherever she goes." However, what you find for yourself may be entirely different than this—and that unexpected surprise is part of the adventure. Still, be careful not to expect too much. Teachers are human as well; don't expect perfection; look instead for a trustworthy source of knowledge; an ally in your journey.

Here are a few tips:

- Look for characteristics you admire. Are they humble? Honest? Good-humored? Do you sense patience as well as practicality in them?
- Do they make grandiose promises or offer vague assurances of miracles—once you pay?
- Do they use an excess of "buzzwords" or currently popular terms? Or do they speak plainly and simply in a way you can understand?
- Do they expect blind obedience, or do they encourage independent thinking? And which is it that you are looking for?
- Do they talk more about *you* than themselves (or their school or their teaching method)?
- Finally, to quote Stephan Bodian one more time, look for someone who embodies "the highest spiritual qualities, such as kindness, patience, equanimity, joy, peace, love, and compassion."

This will not be an easy or entirely painless process. In fact, if you do it right, you will learn as much about yourself and what you're really looking for as you will about the teacher you ultimately choose.

Be patient with yourself and with the world. Take your time. Even the Dalai Lama admitted that Tibetan acolytes could spend years searching for the teacher they needed. It will happen. And even better, you'll learn along the way, even before you've found the teacher you need.

You will ultimately make the practice of meditation—*your* practice of meditation—a unique, highly personal, and very valuable tool in your own personal development.

The Apps of Meditation

Since developing the practice of meditation is, in part, the development of beneficial habits, phone apps can actually have a place in the process for some people. If you're one of those people who enjoys the smartphone interface and uses it easily, consider this (ever-changing) list of phone apps that can help. And check on social media for an updated list. They are presented here in alphabetical order with no specific endorsements given. Shop around, use what works for you and freely fling away the rest.

10% Happier

Free with optional in-app purchases.

An app "designed by skeptics," the goal is to keep meditation from becoming a chore. Includes daily videos and guided meditations, and a wide spectrum of content to help you cope with the day-to-day challenges that create stress.

Aura

Free with optional in-app purchases.

Three to ten minute meditation sessions, nature sounds, mood tracking, thirty second "mindful breathers," a gratitude journal, and an algorithm that personalizes meditations.

Breethe

Free with optional in-app purchases

A five-minute-a-day app compete with a personal mindfulness coach. Guided meditations, inspirational talks, master classes from mindfulness coach Lynne Goldberg, as well as sleep music playlists, nature sounds, and bedtime.

Buddhify

$4.99 for iPhone, $2.99 for Android

More than 200 meditations to help you reduce anxiety and stress, improve your sleep, and manage your emotions, including mindfulness exercises you can practice coping with various everyday challenges, like waking up, eating well, self-care while traveling. Sessions range from three to forty minutes.

Calm

Free with optional in-app purchases

Calming exercises, breathing, sleep stories, and a version that works on the Apple Watch.

Headspace

Free with optional in-app purchases

Guided meditation and mindfulness techniques; sleep music and nature-sound tracks. Headspace builds personalized plans to teach you the essentials of meditation; then you can build your own from there.

Insight Timer

Free with optional in-app purchases

Thousands of guided meditations, with more added every day. Discussion groups and a community feature, as well as music tracks and ambient sounds to inspire, calm, and center.

The Mindfulness App

Free with optional in-app purchases

Mindfulness offers a five day guided practice and introduction and timed-guided or silent meditations from three to thirty minutes in length, as well as personalized meditation options, reminders, and statistics for journaling (an important part of the Jack Dorsey Way).

Sattva

Free with optional in-app purchases

This app is based in the Vedic principles of meditation and features meditations, chants, and mantras delivered by Sanskrit scholars. Includes a meditation journal and playlist to inspire and empower.

Simple Habit

Free with optional in-app purchases

The goal here is stress relief in five minutes a day, to help improve focus, breathe easier, and sleep better.

Stop, Breathe & Think

Free with optional in-app purchases

Meditation recommendations based on your emotions. Techniques offered include short guided meditations, yoga, and acupressure videos. Stop, Breathe & Think allows you to track your mood and your progress, and it offers you an opportunity to check in with yourself every day.

WALKING TO WORK

Jack Dorsey walks to work at least three days a week. It takes him about an hour and fifteen minutes, one way. "I might look a little bit more like I'm jogging than I'm walking," Dorsey says. "It's refreshing ... It's just this one of those take-back moments where you're like, 'Wow, I'm alive!'"

Walking works. It's as simple as that.

In fact, it's hard to find any fitness expert, physician, and generally healthy person at large who doesn't appreciate the benefits of walking on a regular basis. There's not even much debate (at least not anymore) over how much, at a minimum, is good for you. The Department of Health and Human Services recommends at least 150 minutes of "moderate aerobic activity" or seventy-five minutes of "vigorous aerobic activity" or a combination of the two over the course of a week. And you can further amplify the good effects by strength-training exercise of all the major muscle groups at least two times a week (we'll cover that more in the next chapter—the one on Dorsey's dedication to High Intensity Interval Training).

For almost everyone, however, walking alone—if you do it right and often enough—can help with your health. It's a low-impact exercise that can be done for long periods of time, and for many—most, even—it's actually enjoyable.

Walking vs Running: Which is Better?

How does walking compare to running? It doesn't, really; they offer almost entirely different benefits to someone who does either or both...and running really is only appropriate for a smaller subset of people than regular long walks. People with back problems, or with issues around their ankles or knees, should consult a healthcare provider before they commit to running or jogging, and people who are overweight or obese need to be careful about the level of benefit vs investment with jogging. Again, talk to a healthcare professional first.

One advantage of running over many other fitness routines: It tends not to "plateau." Often, you'll see the results from exercise slow down—"flatten out"—after a few weeks or months of consistent use. You have to keep changing routines, switching things up, to get the maximum benefits. So when it comes to walking, this may be the best news of all: There doesn't seem to be any "leveling off" in benefit. The more you walk, the healthier you'll be. It continues to deliver many benefits after many years and many miles without an increase in injury or a decrease in results.

But *is* one better than the other? John Ford, a physiologist who runs a fitness center in New York, says that the two activities offer very different advantages that don't need to be compared. "Running, due to larger muscle recruitment, greater forces exerted and faster motion capability, will always have the proverbial leg up on walking. With that being said, walking is a really good form of exercise and can help you reach your fitness and weight-loss goals."

THE JACK DORSEY WAY

So it's really not a "versus" situation at all. There is plenty to be gained from walking *or* running regularly; it's not "either/or." Jack Dorsey prefers the lower-impact, longer-term commitment of walking to work as part of his regular routine; you may prefer that as well or want to include regular jogging or running as part of your plan, too. But the fact is, almost anyone can benefit from Jack Dorsey's approach, if it's tailored to their individual needs, goals, and lifestyle.

The Proven Benefits of Walking

There are plenty, including:

Walking helps you lose weight and keep weight off. This one may seem obvious, but it's certainly a happy benefit for those who walk regularly. Not only does walking improve muscle tone overall, it improves your body's response to insulin, which can help reduce the most hated of all body fat: belly fat. And it doesn't have to be a huge amount of walking. Moderate weight loss is one of the first and best results of a walking program. Ariel Iasevoli, a personal trainer at Crunch Gyms in New York City, recently told an interviewer with MSN, "Daily walking increases metabolism by burning extra calories *and* by preventing muscle loss, which is particularly important as we get older. One of my clients reduced her body fat by 2 percent in just one month by walking home from work each day, which was just under a mile."

Walking in intervals is one of the secrets to weight reduction. The basic strategy: Warm up for three minutes, then spend twenty-five minutes alternating between a minute of fast walking and a minute of brisk walking (about half the speed of your fast walk). Then end with a two-minute cool-down. Michele Staten, a walking coach and author of *Walk Your Way to Better Health,* explains that interval walking cranks up your "afterburn"—the calories you burn after your walk is officially over. But whatever approach you take, regular walking equals weight loss.

Walking helps prevent or manage high blood pressure and blood sugar (aka type 2 diabetes). Whether it's the American Diabetes, researchers at major universities, or almost anyone who treats (or suffers from) hypertension or type 2 diabetes, they all can agree that walking helps prevent these chronic conditions, helps to regulate them if you have them, and helps in the continuing battle to keep them from getting worse. Just one example: researchers at the University of Boulder Colorado and the University of Tennessee found that regular walking lowered blood pressure by as much as eleven points and may reduce the risk of stroke by 20 to 40 percent. You can check the resources page to find some examples of the studies that back that claim up.

Walking lowers the risk of heart disease. It's all part of the same package—which makes sense, since it's all part of the same body. Walking for almost everyone reduces the chance of having a heart attack or chronic heart disease. Just one example: a 2002 study published in *The New England Journal of Medicine*—and this, too, has been backed up by countless others—tells us that that those who walk thirty

THE JACK DORSEY WAY

or more minutes five or more days a week had a *30 percent lower* risk of cardiovascular disease, compared with those who did not walk regularly. And a recent study published in *Chronic Respiratory Disease* showed that walking may help patients with chronic obstructive pulmonary disease.

The American Heart Association agrees. They recommend at least 150 minutes (that's two and a half hours) of moderate intensive activity every week—basically half an hour a day, five days a week.

Almost half of all adults in the United States have some type of cardiovascular disease. It is the number one cause of death in the U.S., and its ugly stepsister, stroke, is the fifth most common cause of death. You can lower that by as much as *one-third* with just half an hour of walking, five days a week. That's all. That's *it*.

Walking may even help you live longer. This claim is a little harder to pin down, but there is growing evidence that walking—in fact, increased physical activity in general, with walking at the center of the strategy—reduces overall mortality risk, regardless of age, sex, and your fitness level when you begin. A study in the *Journal of the American Geriatrics Society* showed that adults between the ages of seventy and ninety who were physically active lived longer than those who weren't. Scientists at the Swedish School of Sport and Health Sciences in Stockholm examined the health records of over 316,000 adults from Sweden who had their first occupational health screening from 1995 to 2015. They calculated maximal oxygen intake (how much oxygen the lung and heart provide to the muscles during exercise), and found that the more you move around, the higher your oxygen intake will be—and that's a good thing for your muscles, your blood, and your brain. They also looked at overall mortality from cardiovascular events and found that people who increase their activity live longer, healthier lives.

And again, it doesn't have to be a strenuous or complicated undertaking. Dr. Elin Ekblom-Bak, the author of the study, said at the time that, "People think they have to start going to the gym and exercising hard to get fitter. But for most people, just being more active in daily life—taking the stairs, exiting the metro a station early, cycling to work—is enough to benefit health since levels are so low to start with. The more you do, the better."

Walking helps with arthritis and joint pain. Researchers publishing in *Arthritis Research & Therapy* reported that high-intensity interval walk training can help improve immune function in older adults with rheumatoid arthritis. And because regular walking helps improve your range of motion and mobility by increasing blood flow to tense areas, as well as strengthening the muscles around your joints, it can help with all sorts of joint pain. A study in the *American Journal of Preventive Medicine* asked adults who were older than forty-nine years of age who were suffering from lower-body joint pain to walk for an hour each week...and once again, the participants who stuck with their walking routine reported better mobility.

Walking helps trigger improvements in mood, state of mind, and even creativity. This may be the best benefit of all. There's a large body of evidence that shows that regular walking actually *modifies your nervous system* and makes you feel more tranquil and less hostile. One study found that just twelve minutes of walking resulted in an increase in joviality, vigor, attentiveness, and self-confidence versus the same time spent sitting. And that applies to creative output as well. One study from Stanford University found that walking increased creative output by an average of 60 percent. According to the study, "walking opens up the free flow of ideas, and it is a simple and robust solution to the goals of increasing creativity and increasing physical activity." Other studies have reported measurable improvement in memory, the prevention of the deterioration of brain cells as we age, and positive effects on anxiety and depression.

Walking will help you sleep better at night. It's a pretty well-accepted fact that exercise boosts the effects of the "sleep" hormone called *melatonin*, but those positive effects aren't restricted to strenuous exercise. A recent study from the journal *Sleep* focused on postmenopausal women who performed light to moderate intensity physical activity and compared them to another group who were sedentary. The results proved what we already knew; the "walkers" had longer, deeper, higher-quality sleep, and walking also helped reduce pain and stress, which can disturb sleep as well.

The list goes on and on. Regular walking—as little as half an hour, five days a week—can do all of the above, and much more—everything from improving balance and coor-

dination, and increasing bone and muscle strength, to helping with digestion, and even preventing or reducing varicose
veins. There's no reason *not* to start walking, whether you do
it the way Jack Dorsey does, out in nature, or just around your
own neighborhood.

What Do We Mean By "Walking"?

Let's be clear, we're not talking about "power walking" or jogging. Just a brisk walk will do the trick. But there are some good
techniques to get the most out of your walking time.

> **Posture and Purpose.** Pay attention to the "brisk" part of
> "brisk walk." This isn't a leisurely stroll; you're doing this
> for a *reason*, so you need to *focus*. That doesn't mean you
> have to break a sweat to "prove" you're burning calories, but
> you *do* want to pay attention to your posture and keep your
> movements *purposeful*. This includes:

- Keep your head up. Look forward, not at your feet or
  the ground right in front of you.
- Relax your neck, shoulders, and back. Tensing up will
  only hurt later.
- Swing your arms freely. Maybe bend the elbow little.
  You can even pump your arms if you want, but you
  don't have to make a spectacle of yourself.
- Keep your stomach muscles slightly tightened.
- Keep your back straight, not arched forward or backward.
- Practice a "rolling gait"—from heel to toe, heel to toe.
  No clomping or flat-footing.

Warm up, cool down, stretch. Remember that your body is, in one way, a machine made of meat and bone, and it deserves to be well-treated. So warm up first: Walk slowly for five to ten minutes and let your body prepare itself for exercise. At the end of your walk, slow down for another five to ten minutes to avoid cramping and after-the-fact muscle aches. Do a little gentle stretching, before and/or after, to further invite your muscles and joints to the party. You'll thank yourself later.

Get the right gear. Choosing the right shoes is important, but the rest of your clothing is important, too. Keep it comfortable; dress for the weather. And obviously if you're walking near dawn or sunset, and especially at night, wear bright colors. And don't be afraid of reflective tape on your shoes, wrists, or legs. Better to look geeky than invisible at the worst possible time.

What route or routine works for you? The old cliché is that the only exercise (or diet) plan that works is the one you'll actually stick with. So take some time for a serious self-check here. Some people prefer to take the same safe, secure, and familiar route every day. Others prefer variety. Some want to walk *to* somewhere, like the farmer's market or the bookstore (preferably not a fast food joint or a pizza place). Some even prefer to walk inside a local mall to avoid any issues with the weather. Some like to walk with a partner; others prefer to fly solo.

Figure out what works for you…and be honest. There are no wrong answers. Think about what you'd look forward to doing, not just this week or this month, but all year long and the year after that. Think about what time of day and days of the week really work for you. If you have family obligations (like getting the kids off to school) or employment issue (like you *have* to be at work at eight in the morning, no matter what), take that into account…but try and find a free half hour five days a week that you can consistently dedicate to a walk. Don't fall into the "I'll find a time" trap, because after the first few weeks, if you're like every other new walker on earth…you won't.

Jack Dorsey, we know, prefers *outside* to *inside* and to walk to a specific place—his work. But even if that's possible for you…is it something you *want* to do, that's your preference? Think about how quickly you'll get bored, or how easy it will be to make excuses when the time changes or the weather gets bad. And once again: test, measure, and commit.

Set realistic goals. We've already talked about the basic goal: at least half an hour a day, five days a week. But keep in mind that doesn't *have* to be half an hour in one chunk. If your busy day just doesn't make that possible, three ten-minute "bouts" can provide almost the same level of benefit. It all adds up. And even if you don't make the full half hour every day, *anything* is always better than *nothing*. Remind yourself that it's okay to start slow, especially if you haven't been exercising for a while. You can always increase your commitment over time. Maybe start with fifteen minutes, work up to twenty, then move upwards and onwards.

In short, come up with a plan you can stick to, not some unrealistic heaven-high goal you just won't be able to reach.

Track your progress. Keeping a written or digital record of your daily performance can make you more accountable *and* give you all-important moments to celebrate. Your measurement can be time-based, where you simply keep track of how many minutes you walked each day. Or you can use a watch or pedometer to keep track of how many steps you take, or the distance you walked. And you can do your tracking with a phone app or in a journal you keep in the pocket of your running clothes—it doesn't matter how you do it. What *does* matter is that you keep some kind of permanent record, not just rely on your memory, and that you use it as a tool to keep motivated, to congratulate yourself for your milestones (one week, one month, one hundred miles—whatever!)…and to keep moving forward. Literally.

…and don't beat yourself up. This is super-important: *Know that you will fail,* at least a little bit. As your "honeymoon" with walking (and every/any other part of the Jack Dorsey Way) ends, there will be days when your schedule, the weather, an emergency, or even your health will interfere and you just won't make your goal, no matter how reasonable it is—you won't walk five days out of seven, or you'll have to cut a couple of days short and quit after twenty minutes.

It's okay. Perfection is not the goal here; *consistency* is. And the worst thing you can do for your long-term health and happiness is to beat yourself up after a week (or even multiple weeks!) of not reaching your goals. It will just make it that much harder to get back on the horse. So be honest about what pushed you off the plan, work to fix that (if it's fixable), and then begin again. Mark all that in your journal, so you can see your progress as you go.

Now get walking.

Indoors vs Outdoors:
the eternal treadmill controversy

When it comes to walking, there's one question that gets asked more than any other: *Can I do it on a treadmill?*

Certainly that's not the choice that Jack Dorsey made. He has chosen to take longer walks—seventy-five minutes or more—a couple of days a week, instead of shorter walks more often. He's chosen to walk *to* a place—his work—rather than on a course or around his neighborhood. And he's decided to walk outside rather than inside.

The benefits of outdoor walking are fairly obvious. For one, you can avoid distractions like phone and TV screens, unexpected visitors or interruptions. You can drink in the tranquility of the outdoor world—even a busy urban environment—and that will certainly improve your state of mind. And of course walking outside increases your exposure to Vitamin D, the one nutrient we derive directly from the sun, and the one that Americans actually don't get enough of (see our chapter on Vitamin Supplements).

But for some people, outdoor walking simply isn't practical. And they may own or have access to a treadmill, or already belong to a gym.

At base, *walking is walking.* If you're getting the exercise, you're getting many of the benefits regardless of where or how you get the walking done. But make no mistake: You can't just set the treadmill at 3.5 and zone out for half an hour watching your favorite show. Not if you expect to see major results.

More treadmills give you many, *many* options for setting speed, incline, and intervals. Take advantage of that. Make it an *interesting* walk for your body, not just another trudge.

The fact is, you burn more calories by switching it up—repeatedly raising and lowering the heart rate, as opposed to keeping it going at one steady rate, whether that rate is high or low. That tends to happen naturally when you're walking outdoors, whether it's inclines along your route or the need to vary your pace when you come to stop signs or busy streets. So if you want to simulate the calorie burn of an outdoor walk, consider these strategies:

Alter the level of incline. Adjusting the incline on a treadmill can increase the benefits of your "walk" by demanding more from your body. The higher you set the incline, the more energy your body is forced to use, which burns more calories. Now, don't go *too* far. If you've set the pace or incline so aggressively you have to hang on to stay upright, you're gone too far. All that does is reduce the muscle engagement. So be challenging, but don't go crazy.

Try Intervals. Just as you would in an outdoor world walk, start with five minutes at a comfortable speed, no incline. Then try increasing it a small amount—say, 5 percent—for three to five minutes, then go back to a "level playing field" for a minute or two. Repeat this cycle three to five times, and see how you feel. And you can add difficulty by increasing the length of each interval *before* you move on to a higher incline or a faster pace.

Consider Adding Weights. While walking on an incline, you might try working out a bit with dumbbells—shoulder presses or jab—that can help tone your upper body and increase your calorie burn as you walk. You can even hop off the treadmill and try some weighted squats, jumping jacks, or sit-ups. And if you don't have fancy dumbbells around, books in a backpack or water in a jug with a handle can work just as well

Even without the spiritual, psychological, or nutritional advantages of the outdoors, there's nothing wrong with a treadmill instead of a walk to work (like Dorsey) or anywhere else outside. Again: anything is better than nothing at all!

Choosing a Walking Shoe

Walking doesn't require a lot of fancy equipment or clothing...but you *do* need a good pair of shoes. So take some time to test and choose the shoe that's best for you and your situation.

Measure twice, buy once. Remember, your feet change as you grow up and grow old. Your tendons, ligaments, and muscles stretch. They can get wider and longer after years of use; the fatty pads that line the bottom of your feet can get thinner. Assume nothing: Whenever you buy a new pair of shoes, measure your feet; don't rely on your memory of Way Back When. And measure *both* your feet. If one is larger than the other, go with the larger size.

Give in to the Pain. Now is not the time to be brave. If you have regular or chronic pain in your back, knees, or heels, you'll want a more supportive shoe that provides extra cushioning under the heel. Bunions or pain in your big toe from arthritis, or gout, or numbness or tingling from diabetic neuropathy are also factors you should take into account.

What Will the Weather Be? Don't just think about today's forecast. Think about the future: Rain? Snow? Ice? You'll want these shoes to support you, structurally and personally, the whole year 'round. So think about the treads, the traction, and whether they need to be waterproof or not.

The AARP, of all people, has a handy (or footy!) list of shoe-buying tips to keep in mind. Here's a summary:

THE JACK DORSEY WAY

- **Buy the right size…but *don't* go by the size marked on the shoe.** Sizes can vary by style, brand, and even the country in which the shoes were manufactured. Pay attention to how they feel on your feet, not by the numbers.

- **Shape matters.** Choose shoes that fit the shape of your feet—wide, narrow, long-toed, whatever.

- **Wiggle your toes.** The space at the end of your shoe where your toes go is called, not surprisingly, the "toe-box," and it should be spacious enough that you can freely wiggle your toes, but not so loose that your foot actually slides forward. It may take a bit of attention to get the right size and shape. Also, allow at least three-eighths of an inch from the tip of your longest toe to the tip of your shoes. Basically, you should be able to push the tip of your index finger between the tip of your longest toe and the end of the shoe.

- **Stand up. Walk around.** Make sure that you're not feeling uncomfortable pressure on the side *or* the bottom of your feet, as well as noting any pressure or crowding at the toe and heel. And walk all around the store. Take as long as you want. Remember, you'll be wearing these for long intervals, so you want them to feel good after five or ten minutes, not just after thirty seconds.

- **Don't expect your shoes to "stretch out."** They won't. Obviously there's always a little stiffness, especially in the sole, but if the shoe feels too tight when you put it on in the store, it's not going to loosen a day or a week later.

- **Buy your shoes at the end of the day**. This may sound strange, but it's true: Everyone's feet swell (not smell, *swell*) as the day goes on, and it's important that the shoes you buy fit comfortably even when your feet are at their naturally largest state.

HIGH-INTENSITY INTERVAL TRAINING (HIIT)

**When Dorsey doesn't walk to work,
he does high-intensity intervals on an exercise
bike and seven-minute workouts. "I don't have
a personal trainer. I don't go to a gym."**

J ack Dorsey's commitment to health is an every-day (though far from everyday) thing, and on the days he doesn't walk to work, he doesn't lay back. Quite the opposite, he leans forward, with a commitment to the highly popular and highly effective fitness regimen called "High-Intensity Internal Training." It is a program that focuses on twelve specific exercises using only his body weight, a chair, and a wall, packing a huge amount of beneficial activity into just a few minutes.

What's just as important is that HIIT grew out of scientific research aimed at creating the optimal workout. The goal: to create the molecular changes in thin muscles similar to hours of running, bike-riding, or weight-lifting.

Briefly put—just as it was in the article that started it all, originally published in the American College of Sport Medicine's *Health and Fitness Journal* in 2013—HIIT is simple and straightforward. The exercises are:

- Jumping jacks
- Wall sit
- Push-ups
- Abdominal crunches
- Step-up onto a chair
- Squats
- Triceps dip on a chair
- Plank
- High knees, running in place
- Alternating lunges
- Push-ups with rotation
- Side plank, each side

Each exercise is performed for thirty seconds, followed by a ten-second rest, for a total of about seven minutes of work. However, the plan suggests three reeditions of the entire process, for a total of twenty-one minutes or so.

The key to HIIT, however, is the *interval*. The idea is to perform extremely intensive exercises followed by brief periods of recovery. The sequence of exercises is important as well, so the work focuses on the large muscles in the upper body alternating with those in the lower body. This way, the unexercised muscles have a chance to rest as the focus moves on, only to return for another round in a few minutes. This strategy also explains why the exercises should be performed in rapid succession, and why the intensity should actually make you a little uncomfortable. It's hard, but it's *fast*.

Even though the specific routine seemed to appear overnight, it has actually been used in various forms by dedicated athletes for hundreds of years. And its acceptance and popularity seemed to explode just as quickly, for one simple reason: It actually *works* for many people, and there's science to back up the results. Over the years since its introduction, multiple research papers have proved its potential to increase cardiorespiratory endurance, increase muscle mass, control blood press, and speed the loss of body fat that "steady state" cardio exercise can.

Is HIIT Better Than "Steady State" Exercise?

The theory all along has been that working very hard, then resting, then working hard again, back and forth, results in more calories being burned up in less time.

And the research seems to back that up. If, for instance, you run on a treadmill for thirty minutes and compare the calorie burn to doing thirty minutes of steady state cardio, you will burn more calories. The same seems to apply according to comparisons between HIIT and steady-state weight training. But there's more to weight loss and good health than just calorie burn. In fact, Jack Dorsey's combination of walking and HIIT is a good approach; you get the benefit of both in a flexible plan that can last a lifetime.

Here are some of the unique benefits of making HIIT part of your plan:

- HIIT not only burns more calories during the workout itself, but studies show you
- burn more calories for about two hours *after* exercise— something that doesn't happen with steady-state cardio.
- People who commit to HIIT actually like it and tend to stay with it longer. Studies have shown that people enjoy HIIT far more than continued moderate-intensive workouts, perhaps because of its relative simplicity and how little time it takes. Whatever the reason, it's a keeper.
- HIIT workouts can boost your endurance, and that benefit will carry over into your other moderate-intensity activities like sports and walking.
- HIIT may offer even greater cardiovascular benefits than moderate-intensive workouts. The theory, still being confirmed, is that HIIT increases the flexibility and elasticity of your arteries and veins better than "normal" aerobic exercise. Many believe that it's not only safe, but superior to other forms of exercise for people with coronary artery disease.

How to get started?

Thanks to YouTube, anyone can learn how to do anything; and that includes learning about HIIT. If you'd rather the in-person experience, you can take a local call from a trained fitness instructor—even just once or twice—to get the hang of it. And even Jack Dorsey himself uses an app to prompt him, time his work, and keep track of his commitment. We've included a very partial list of some of the most popular HIIT apps below.

It's not hard to get started, but it *is* hard to stick with, especially in the early days as your body is getting used to the demands and rewards of high-intensive interval training. Take a good long look at it; talk to some people who've been working the plan for a while, and see if it makes sense as an adjunct to our walking programs. Either one alone offers great benefits, and so the two together can work miracles.

Ten Best HIIT Workout Apps for Fitness Enthusiasts

High-Interval Intensity Training (HIIT) is perfectly designed for the phone app. Here are some of the most popular apps around as of 2019, including Seven, the one that Jack Dorsey uses. Do some research, get some recommendations…and get to it!

Flit—Interactive fitness (Flit)

Free with in-app purchases.

100 different workouts by real trainers.

Freeletics—Workout & Fitness. Body Weight App (Freeletics)

Free with in-app purchases.

Thousands of HIIT workouts, 24/7 fitness advice, ten- to thirty-minute workout plans, articles and blogs.

HIIT & Cardio Workout By Fitify (Martin Mazanec)

Free with in-app purchases.

More than ninety bodyweight exercises in four different workout programs; audio and video tutorials.

Interval Timer—HIIT Training (Appxy)

Free with in-app purchases.

A user-friendly, hassle-free app that tracks time for your workout and rest periods alike, recording highs and lows and even pauses when resting.

The J&J Official 7 Minute Workout (Johnson & Johnson Health & Wellness Solutions)

Free.

Seventy-two exercises and twenty-two preset and customizable workouts, from seven to thirty-two minutes available. Video tutorials.

Seconds Pro—Interval Timer (Runloop Ltd.)

$4.99.

Employs an AI to create a personalized program; tracks daily progress; even allow real-time chats and emails for questions. Data-sync with Google Fit. Custom timers, large timer display, music integration. Simple and fun to use.

Seven: 7-Minute Workout (Perigee)

Free with in-app purchases, including club membership.

One of the most popular HIIT apps available, and the one that Jack Dorsey has used. Personalized workout plans tailored to your goals for losing or maintaining weight, getting fit, getting strong, and so forth. Cool instructors like "The Cheerleader" and "The Drill Instructor."

Sworkit Fitness (Sworkit)

Free with in-app purchases.

Guides, workouts plans or build your own customized intervals, and trainer advice.

Workout Trainer: Fitness Coach (Skimble, Inc.)

Free with paid PRO+ membership

Thousands of workouts and custom-made training programs for its users. Trainers who guide you through sharing pictures, videos, and audio tutorials. Variable difficult levels, wearable connectivity, exercise summary logs.

SAUNAS AND ICE BATHS

**Jack Dorsey takes ice baths in the morning
and saunas and ice baths in the evening. "Nothing has
given me more mental confidence than being able to go
straight from room temperature into the cold," he says,
"especially in the morning. Going into an ice-cold tub from
just being warm in bed...unlocks this thing in my mind and
I feel like if I can will myself to do that thing that seems
so small but hurts so much, I can do nearly anything."**

J ack Dorsey is a true believer in the therapeutic value of
hyperthermia and *hypothermia*—the pursuit of health
through exposure to extreme temperatures, both heat
and cold. It's a practice that is almost as old as civilization itself,
especially in cultures where such extremes are a natural part of
the environment. In Scandinavia, as an example, hot-then-cold
activities are a way of life. Many residents of Finland who use
saunas three to five times a week, and claim to live long and
healthier lives because of it, were more healthy and lived longer
than those that never used them.

And devotees of this practice claim it has a vast array of benefits, from relaxation to longer life to treating diabetes.

The basis for these claims are more cultural than scientific, but one thing is clear: there are millions of people that swear by the positive power of the ice bath and/or the sauna, and many people—excepting those with medical conditions that can make these practices dangerous—may find ice bath and saunas stimulating, relaxing, and even enlightening.

Jack Dorsey's approach is a fairly common one: He sits in a barrel sauna set at 220 degrees Fahrenheit, then hops into an ice bath at a temperature in the high thirties, just above freezing, for about three minutes. Then he repeats that process three times, finishing with one more sixty second ice bath. Dorsey uses a small tent-shaped sauna that relies on a near-infrared bulb to provide its heat. Dorsey has said he feels this technology helps him sweat more than a dry sauna, at a much lower temperature (and we will look at the various sauna technologies later in this chapter).

What Do Ice Baths and Saunas Actually Do to Your Body?

There's no question that extreme temperature can have a significant effect on human tissue and physiology. Professional athletes have used ice baths to reduce inflammation and sooth sore muscles for centuries; physical therapists swear by the positive effects of both heat and cold in pain management and healing. Ned Brophy-Williams, an Australian sports scientist and author, told *Fast Company* that an ice bath redirects blood flow "from the peripheral to deep blood vessels, thereby limiting inflammation and swelling and improving venous return." "Improving venous return" means speeding the removal of metabolites and waste products that build up in muscles after strenuous exercise. And many of its proponents gives special value to alternating between ice baths or cold showers and exposure to heat through saunas or immersion—much like Jack Dorsey does.

And there are psychological benefits as well. As Dorsey himself has said, he feels more positive and more energetic after his morning hot/cold routine, and a 2007 survey from the Virginia Commonwealth University School of Medicine, among many others, backs him up. It found evidence that cold showers can help treat depression symptoms, and, if used regularly, might even be more effective than prescription antidepressants. The chief researcher on the project was interviewed for a podcast called *NeuroScene* a few years ago, and said, "The mechanism that can probably explain the immediate mood-lifting effect of immersion in cold water or cold shower is probably the stimulation of the dopaminergic transmission in the mesocorticolimbic and nigrostriatal pathway. There is a lot of research linking these brain areas to depression."

Prolonged exposure to heat affects the body in different but equally profound ways. A sauna can raise the skin temperature to roughly 104 degrees Fahrenheit. As the skin temperature rises, heavy sweating occurs, and the heart rate rises as the body tries to keep itself cool. It is not uncommon to lose about a pint of sweat while spending even a short time in a sauna.

Finally, the combination of the two—a sauna followed by cold immersion—causes your blood vessels to constrict rapidly and as a result, elevate blood pressure and increases blood flow.

The Hoped-For, Widely Claimed Benefits of Ice Baths and Saunas

Here's where things get a little murky. Depending on where you look and who you believe, hyperthermia and hypothermia are credited with a startling array of benefits.

For instance, ice baths are claimed to:

- Stimulate muscular, cardiovascular, and nervous system recovery
- Decrease joint and muscle pain
- Increase alertness and provide more energy
- Improve immune system performance
- Help you sleep better
- Enhance your ability to burn fat
- Improve endurance
- Help with blood sugar control

Heat therapy is credited with a similar list of benefits, including:

- Better skin tone and color—a "glow"
- Muscle relaxation
- Improved circulation
- Stress reduction

- Better sleep
- Enhanced muscle building
- Decreased joint and muscular pain
- Improved cognitive function
- Reduced resting heart rate
- Reduced blood pressure
- Increase in red blood cell count
- And once again, better blood sugar control

...and in both cases, there is a widespread and oft-repeated "benefit" related to "removing toxins from the body" through stress and sweat.

What the Science Says

We'll discuss the "toxins" and "stress" issues separately, but as for some of the other claims:

The "glowing skin" claim has no scientific studies to support it, but it certainly makes sense. That "healthy glow" comes from the opening of your blood vessels after exposure to heat. Very simply, light reflects different off of skin when the blood vessels are open, and most humans perceive this as a characteristic of health.

The relief of muscle soreness is a real thing. Whether it's from injury or a chronic condition like arthritis, there's no question that heat and light humidity make your body feel better. Ask any athlete. This is due primarily to the increased blood circulation, and that's a good thing.

It really doesn't help you lose weight. It's true that a body exposed to the heat and cold of these practices does burn more calories than a body at rest, but you're really looking at calorie expenditure similar to a moderate cardio workout of the same duration. And some small studies looking for other improvements really didn't find any when it came to improvement in heart rate, lactate concentration, or oxygen uptake. And weight loss attributed to the process is pretty standard water-weight loss you could achieve at about the same level through a number of other means.

It may give you more energy, but that's as much psychological and physiological. The whole process does elevate your heart rate and then relax your muscles. Once it's over and you've recovered, you're likely to feel refreshed and more alert than you might without it (as Jack Dorsey himself alludes to in the opening quote). But there's no measurable increase in hours you can work or energy you can expend. By the same token, it will almost certainly help most people sleep better…but then so will any increase in physical activity, like regular walking or High-Intensity Interval Training as described in earlier chapters.

Bottom Line, it might help. After all, a zillion Scandinavians can't be wrong. But don't expect hyperthermia or hypothermia to heal you or prevent disease in any miraculous or measurable way. There's no evidence to support that.

Be careful!

The physiological and psychological benefits of this approach are obvious, if not quite as profound as some think...but as is the case with almost all "healthy lifestyle" advice—it depends on the individual.

Think of it this way: When you plunge into frigid water, from an overheated state or even a normal room-temperature state, your body goes into "cold shock," and that puts a strain on your heart. Blood vessels on the outer part of your body constrict, as they attempt, quite automatically, to retain what body heat remains. Blood shifts to your inner organs as your body tries to keep them warm just a little longer. And that shift-and-shock can be very uncomfortable, though for most healthy people it only lasts a few minutes at most.

However...if you are at high risk of heart disease, the blood vessels in the heart can constrict as well, and that may lead to chest pains or even heart attack or angina. What's more, this sudden "cold shock" triggers the release of adrenaline, our favorite stress hormone, and that surge can trigger an irregular heart rhythm—another risky situation for people with heart issues.

So consider that strain you're putting on your body *before* your take the plunge. This is especially true if:

- You have a history of heart attacks or cardiovascular disease
- You have a family history of stroke
- You have chronic high blood pressure (hypertension)

- You are pregnant or lactating
- You have an implanted electric device like a pacemaker

In any of these cases, you'll want to talk with your healthcare provider before you begin any program that involves extremes of heat and/or cold.

The "Toxin" Myth

As you research the potential for hyperthermia and hypothermia, you will almost certainly run into a great deal of talk about its potential to remove "toxins" from your body. This is a claim that is also made by a wide range of other (often dubious) medical or fitness procedures, "super foods," or folk remedies. However, this notion isn't backed up by any scientific research or even basic biology. It may, in fact, grow from a fundamental misunderstanding of how the human body works.

There's no question that there are toxins in our environment. Every one of us is exposed to and ingests toxins every day—every hour. But over millions of years, the human body has evolved the ability to cleanse itself of those toxins on a continuing and highly efficient basis. We have two organs that are beautifully designed and dedicated to exactly that process: the liver and the kidney.

The misunderstanding comes in when people believe that the kidney and liver operate like the stomach or intestines. It's true, the gastrointestinal tract *can* become "clogged" or blocked with poorly digested material; it can become infected, or in extreme cases even dangerously septic, and it can benefit from a chemical or even mechanical purgation in those cases.

This is not true of the liver or kidney. These organs work in an entirely different way; they do not process food or any substance in the way the stomach or intestine does, and they cannot become clogged or blocked in the same way. Of course they can become less efficient because of disease, abuse, or age, and they can even

---

fail—which leads to serious health problems. But they cannot be and should not be "purged" in any way, nor does any other part of the body contain "toxins" that need to be driven out by any means.

Of course there are exceptions. Mercury, copper, lead, some other heavy metals, as well as actual poisons and toxic chemicals, may need to be removed from the body, but very few of the "alternative" methods we hear about—including extreme heat and cold—can affect these serious issues. They require a doctor's intervention and an entirely different medical approach, like chelation therapy.

Your body is not swimming with toxins. It does not need to be purged. And even if it did, increasing the amount you sweat, in a belief that toxins can be shed through perspiration, simply isn't true.

Some time ago, Dr. Dee Anna Glaser, a dermatology professor at St. Louis University and the president of the International Hyperhidrosis Society, was interviewed as part of an excellent article about sweat and toxins that appeared in *The Atlantic* magazine. You couldn't find a better authority—Dr. Glaser is an expert on "hyperhidrosis," the medical term for "excessive sweating." "In general," she told *The Atlantic*, "sweat can release some toxins and some chemicals, but that is not really sweat's major job. The organs responsible for detoxifying our system are the kidneys and the liver. Those two do such a good job that, really, sweat doesn't need to do that. So, for most people, sweating a lot does not detoxify them at all. Because the kidneys are doing it. Sweat's main job is to keep us cool." Other experts also quoted in *The Atlantic* agreed. Hershel Raff, one of the authors of a standard textbook on human physiology, said, "Sweat contains salt (sodium and chloride) that can represent a large loss of electrolytes with a large volume of sweat (e.g. exercising on a hot day)." Very small amounts of lead, copper, and nickel do appear in sweat, but sauna-level sweating won't remove them. Only far more demanding chelation therapy, undertaken by a medical specialist, can help in those rare cases.

The news, then, is both good and bad (isn't it always?): You don't need to worry nearly as much about toxins in your environment as you may think you do. If you are a relatively healthy human, your liver and kidney are doing an excellent job at keeping those toxins under control in your body, and no amount of sweating or other practices will help that (though there are plenty of ways to hurt it, like drinking alcohol, obesity, or smoking tobacco). The bad news is there are plenty of medical "experts" that will continue to promote the "toxin" myth so they can sell you expensive technologies, procedures, medications, or ingestibles to "cure" you of a problem you don't actually have, or that their magic devices or substances can't really address.

Choosing the Right Sauna

So if you've decided to give the sauna/ice bath approach a try… how do you choose the right sauna (the ice bath or ice shower part is pretty easy!)? A scan of all the websites and options available can be pretty daunting, and we won't attempt to provide you with a *Consumer Reports*-level scan of what's available or recommended. But here are a few basics:

Sauna Types. Basically, saunas come in two varieties: Traditional (employing steam) and Infrared.

Traditional (Steam) is almost always a permanent, indoor facility that uses rocks heated by electricity. Water is thrown onto the hot rocks to create steam. A steam sauna takes about an hour to heat up and can reach a temperature of 160–200 degrees Fahrenheit. A traditional sauna is typically more expensive than other options and uses more electricity.

Infrared saunas come in two flavors: **Far-infrared saunas** use heating elements that mainly emit light in the far-infrared spectrum, but do not penetrate the body as well as Near-infrared light. **Near-infrared saunas** combine heat therapy and light therapy. Infrared saunas take about ten to fifteen minutes to heat up and are about thirty degrees cooler than traditional saunas. Jack Dorsey and others feel they get a better "sweat" from infrared saunas than from traditional steam-based technology.

Wayfair, the online furniture retailer, has an excellent "how-to" on choosing and buying the right sauna for your needs. They—as well as a wide range of other online and brick-and-mortar retailers—can offer everything from tent-like, portable, single-person saunas (rather like the one that Jack Dorsey often uses), through two-person permanent units, all the way to beautifully crafted six-person permanent installations made from cedar. Prices can range from as little as a couple of hundred dollars to more than six thousand.

There is also a less expensive "portable" option. These portable units are made of durable, moisture-resistant material and include a chair for you to sit on; they are zipped up around your body while your head remains exposed. The heating elements may be steam or infrared light; both versions can be plugged into a wall outlet.

As you're making your decision, pay attention to the **type of heater** your sauna uses. **Ceramic heaters** heat up more quickly than other technologies, but they tend to be more delicate. **Carbon fiber** heaters are slower but more durable and more energy-efficient than ceramic and usually offer a more even heat distribution.

EMF ratings are important, too. Infrared saunas emit electromagnetic fields (EMF). Ceramic heaters typically emit a lower EMF than carbon heaters, and saunas that have a combination of the two types of heaters emit the lowest EMF. Experts generally recommend that you keep your EMF exposure under three milligauss. Be sure the sauna you choose has passed ETL certification, and you can be assured it's safe without further inquiry.

Most permanent saunas are made from cedar—fragrant, rot-resistant, and antifungal. Though it is expensive, it's also very durable. Hemlock is popular as well, and though it is not naturally rot-resistant or antifungal, Wayfair tells us it is hypoallergenic, scentless, knot-free, and is not easily scratched or damaged.

Finally, before you order your dream sauna, do a little planning. Ask and answer the following questions:

- Are you going to install it yourself, or ask for professional help?
- Where are you going to place it—indoors, or outdoors, and exactly where?
- Do you have the necessary water and electrical hook-ups required, or will some "prep" work be required? (Most saunas work with the standard 110–120 volt

outlets, but some require heavier-duty wiring. Double-check before you buy!)

- If you're opting for one of the larger models, do you want a bench?
- Do you want the capability to play music inside? (Speakers and mp3 players are available)
- Will you want to use your phone inside the sauna? (Bluetooth compatibility is available.)
- Will you want or need a timer to regulate your time in the sauna?
- Finally, be aware that a sauna, like an outdoor pool, requires a significant amount of maintenance even when it's not in use. Take the periodic washing and weather protection commitments into account when you're choosing both the size and location of your sauna. (For instance, if you opt for the traditional sauna, you need to reset the rocks in the heater once a year!)

EATING ONE MEAL A DAY AND FASTING ON WEEKENDS

From Monday through Thursday, Dorsey only eats dinner, usually between 6:30 and 9 p.m. "During the day, I feel so much more focused...and the time back from breakfast and lunch allowed me to focus more on what my day is." Then he will skip dinner on Friday and fast until Sunday evening.

Jack Dorsey is a big believer in a health trend that has become very popular and continues to grow. It goes under the general rubric of "intermittent fasting," and he—like many other people—has broken it into two components: eating one meal a day Monday through Friday, and then fasting entirely on Saturday and Sunday.

We're going to examine both approaches at once, since they touch on so many of the same issues. Let's begin with the practice that's become so popular it even has its own acronym: OMAD, for "One Meal A Day."

OMAD: The Basics

There are YouTube videos, websites, bestselling diet books, and a rising wave of crazy claims relating to OMAD and its possible—*possible*—health benefits. It's not surprising; fasting as a spiritual and physical discipline (and a harsh reality) has been with us for as long as there have been humans, across almost all cultures. Asian mystics practiced it, Socrates and Plato advocated for it, but integrating it into twenty-first century life is a relatively new development.

Let's get the definition out of the way first:

One Meal A Day allows you to eat a single meal every twenty-four hours. You may drink calorie-free liquids during the other twenty-three hours, but no solid food.

For some reason, most OMAD proponents seem to take their meals in the evening, just as Jack Dorsey does, though there's no known, clinically verified advantage to one time of day over another.

What you eat during that one daily meal is open-ended; every "expert" in the field seems to have a different opinion (and all too often, a different related product to sell). Dorsey himself sticks to fairly traditional choices: fish, chicken, or steak with a salad or side of vegetables, and often a dessert of berries or chocolate. But you'll notice he's neither vegan nor vegetarian, and he seems to avoid binge-eating in general and junk food in particular. Other proponents differ wildly, on both sides of the spectrum. There is no "standard" OMAD diet.

Why OMAD?

Among the most commonly repeated benefits of OMAD, you'll hear that eating one meal a day can help you:

- Lose weight
- Increase mental acuity
- Improve your mood and outlook
- Control blood sugar, cholesterol, and high blood pressure
- Save money
- Save time
- Develop self-discipline
- Sleep better
- Live longer

How many of these claims are true? An excellent question. We'll tackle each one separately as we go and talk about the risks as well as the benefits related to OMAD and intermittent fasting, too. First, ask yourself: How many of these benefits are even measurable? The answer is not many. And how many *have* been measured, considering how recently this new fitness strategy has become popular? The answer is even fewer. There's still much investigative work to be done, and even when the results of ongoing research are in, many of your decisions concerning OMAD and what variation you choose to pursue will be based on your own personal feelings and circumstances, not just the facts.

One thing, however, is clear: Jack Dorsey is not alone in his dedication to the ideas that are central to intermittent fasting in all its forms.

How Hunger (and Eating) Works

Before we dig too deep into the subcategories and variations of intermittent fasting, let's spend some time talking about the basics of *eating, hunger,* and *food.*

There was a time, not so long ago, when scientists thought they understood the relatively simple biological bases of hunger. For a while, there was great hope that we could learn to control or simply block a particular hormone (that is, a set of chemicals that carry messages from one part of the body to another) called *leptin,* and in doing so, we could control weight gain and overeating better than any diet or existing "diet pills" (that were largely limited to reformulated and repackaged amphetamines).

It turned out that blocking or reducing leptin production didn't really work very well. People still overate and still gained weight, and over the last couple of decades, research has shown us that the whole internal process of eating is far more complicated than we believed. There's much more to controlling it than just throwing a single chemical switch. Vastly different areas of the brain are involved; psychological factors, behavioral issues, and genetics all play important roles as well. And today, nutritionists and scientists generally agree that there are at least six hormones that influence hunger alone, and three signifi-

THE JACK DORSEY WAY

cant influences that affect an individual's eating patterns. The three factors are:

- Hunger
- Satiety
- Perseverance

Hunger is the easy one. We all know what hunger feels like. It is the body telling the brain that it needs fuel. It's that hollowness, that compulsion, that *need* to eat. But how we express those feelings of hunger, how we respond to them, is filtered through an array of learned behaviors, physiological needs, and real-world issues that deeply affect what we actually do when we feel that hunger coming on.

At the same time, there's *satiety,* a distinctly different, though related, issue. This is the sensation of feeling full, feeling *satisfied* with the food you've just consumed. This, too, is controlled at least in part by hormones, but it is equally susceptible to the lessons you were taught as a child. Were you a member of the Clean Plate Club? Do you not feel *satisfied* if there is still food on the table, waiting to be eaten? What eating habits do you have (like snarfing a full bag of chips in front of the TV) that play into satiety?

Finally, there's *perseverance,* pronounced "purr-SEHV-ur-unce" in this usage. This is the least known or fully understood of the factors. It has to do with *focus*—thinking about food, concentrating on food, *obsessing* on food, even when you are not particularly hungry and are feeling satiated. Basically, even when you're fed and full, you find that you can't stop thinking about *food*—about your next meal, or what other people are eating at that moment, or even a random image or smell that triggers a whole cascade of emotions and compulsions. An entirely different set of brain chemicals and behaviors, as well as the constant barrage of food-marketing (for junk food and for healthy alternatives alike) can influence perseverance as well, so simply blocking a single chemical that only attacks one part of the hunger/eating process simply won't do the trick.

What's more, your body is wired to keep you eating as much as you can, as often as you can. There is a scientifically verified process called *weight defense,* something our bodies have been doing "for" us since we first evolved, that often works against us as we try to take control of our eating patterns. Check out the box in this chapter to learn more about weight defense.

All of these issues come into play when you start making major changes in how much you eat and when you eat it—and shifting from three meals a day to one, and to two days with no food at all, has to be considered *major*.

The Secret Six-Word Secret to Weight Loss

Given this complexity and decades of research and experimentation, it's become tragically clear: The answer to losing weight and/or keeping weight off isn't really a matter of a single strategy, medication, or diet. However, all that research *has* revealed two central facts:

- No one diet plan or approach is superior to another; plenty of strategies succeed at helping *some* people control their eating, but nothing helps *everyone*.

- Virtually all of the most long-lasting and effective approaches do share one common thread—a core concept that can be expressed in six words:

Eat Less

Eat Better

Exercise More

Like all great ideas, it's easy to express and very difficult to follow through on a regular basis. But it truly is that simple.

Eat Less is not simply a matter of controlling your calories (we'll get into that a little later on). That's part of it, sure. The fancy name for it is *portion control,* but finding the exact set of tricks and tools that make it possible for you, the individual *you,* is a real challenge.

The simple fact of the matter, however, is that Americans— and most Western nations—simply *eat too much.* We consume far more food-mass—high- and low-calorie, low-fat and high-fat, high-protein and no-protein, solid and liquid—than we need to on a daily basis, and OMAD and intermittent fasting are two ways to deal with that issue directly—maybe even brutally.

Eat Better is open to wide interpretation, but here, too, there are some core principles that virtually everyone agrees on. More fruits and vegetables. Less heavily processed food that's loaded with salt or saturated fats. Little or no added sugar. More fish and less (or maybe no?) red meat, though vegetarianism and its more extreme cousins present challenge and concerns all their own. We can rage and worry over everything from gluten to GMOs to all around that, but truly, the work of generations of health professionals have told us there are many paths to paradise.

Exercise More is probably the most overlooked element of those words. For one thing, many people are actively repelled by the idea of "exercise"—going to a gym, straining with weights or machines, sweating to the oldies (or newbies), *hurting* yourself to lose weight, gaining muscle, getting healthy. It's become such an unpopular word, in fact, that many dietitians, nutritionists, and trainers avoid the word entirely now, in favor of a softer and more accurate word: *activity.* But the reality behind it is that it doesn't much matter what diet plan or eating pattern you follow; if you're not increasing your activity to burn calories and build muscle mass, you're far less likely to lose anything but a few pounds of water weight.

Jack Dorsey (as usual) has figured this out. His multi-part strategy includes activity (his walks and HIIT regimen) *and* a plan that both reduces his food intake and increases its quality. However you manage the details of your own plan, incorporating both those elements—elements that embody the Six Words—gives you a far better chance of working for you.

From "Diet" to "Eating Pattern"

Even the word "diet" is falling out of favor. "Diet" implies a lot of rules and restrictions, a rigid plan you *have to follow*, every day, or you will "fail;" and nobody wants to be a *failure.* That's the single biggest problem with many of the weight loss and eating plans that exist now; it's not that many of them aren't effective, in the short term at least. It's that the abandonment rate is *huge*. Here again, dieticians, nutritionists, doctors, and trainers agree: *Consistency* is the key to losing weight, keeping it off, or never gaining it in the first place. If you stop thinking of it as a "win/loss," as a "success/failure," the chances that you'll stick with your decision and thereby change your life increase greatly. Therefore, try to think of your relationship to food and eating as a series of *patterns,* as opposed to *rules.*

One Meal A Day, and in the larger, context intermittent fasting in general, is a classic case of "pattern" over "diet." Each individual can choose when and how to implement the pattern—what foods to eat and when, how often to commit to a fast—and since there are no "rules" to begin with, there don't have to be "cheat days" (another term that implies dishonesty and failure). If you start from that place, it's much easier to forgive yourself for momentary slip-ups or distractions and to re-commit to a pattern.

Mindfulness

What it really comes down to—with OMAD, intermittent fasting, veganism, and all the other various eating patterns—is building a personal and permanent state of *mindfulness.* These are all strategies designed to help you—sometimes even *force* you—to think about what (and when and why) you are putting a particular food into your body.

As we'll see, committing to OMAD and weekend fasting (or for almost any other element in the Jack Dorsey Way) requires *thought* as well as *action.* It demands a level of awareness that can be rewarding in itself, but it also is a test of just how serious you are about changing your life. There's nothing in the Jack Dorsey plan that is a "quick fix"—nothing that you can do once and be done—no "fix and forget." It's the *intentional* commitment to a set of *patterns*—eating, exercise, behavioral *patterns*—that can change your life for the better. It's not something that just *happens* to you; it's something you have to *make* happen.

So Back to Business: Will OMAD and Weekend Fasting Help Me?

The answer to the question is the most annoying (and truthful) answer you can hear to any question: *It depends.* Taking the issues one at a time...

Will it help me lose weight? Most likely...yes. If you're only eating one meal a day, it would be almost impossible to consume as much, purely in volume, as you formerly consumed when you ate three meals a day (and snacks! Don't forget snacks!). So purely on the basis of caloric intake, you'll probably lose some weight.

A growing array of scientific studies back this up. In fact, a systematic review of forty separate studies found that intermittent fasting triggered a weight loss of seven to eleven pounds over a period of ten weeks—and this covered participants of varying ages and body types, from old to young and from slightly overweight to clinically obese.

There's also evidence that OMAD and intermittent fasting help with sleep, so here again, logic intervenes: If you're awake fewer hours a day, then you're expending less energy and taking in fewer calories than you did pre-OMAD.

The real question, however, is does OMAD or intermittent fasting allow you to lose weight *faster* or can you lose *more* than through an old-fashioned, continuous calorie-restriction diet? And on that front, it looks as if this answer is somewhere between "no" and "we don't know yet."

That same forty-study review mentioned above also showed that dropout rates were about the same between traditional diet plans and intermittent fasting; there was also no significant difference in the amount of weight lost or in BMI; there might have been a slightly greater sense of appetite in the intermittent fasting group—essentially, they felt more hungry more often than the traditional group—but that was about it.

So if you're looking for a way to lose more weight quicker than what you've experienced with more traditional calorie-restricting diet plans...OMAD and intermittent fasting aren't going to help.

Will it help increase my mental acuity? Possibly. There is *some* evidence that fasting might improve mental acuity. Johns Hopkins neuroscience professor Mark Mattson, senior investigator at the National Institute on Aging's Laboratory of Neurosciences, has shown intermittent fasting can help "ward off neurodegenerative diseases like Alzheimer's and Parkinson's while at the same time improving memory and mood."

"There's a lot of evidence from animals that fasting—*intermittent* fasting—can enhance cognition," he said in an excellent article on wellandgood.com, "and there's quite a bit of info emerging on what might be the underlying cellular and molecular mechanisms—the signals, the hormones, and the neurotransmitters involved." And interestingly, this isn't just about being sharper when you're hungry—not at all. Dr. Mattson and other researchers around the world are looking specifically at intermittent fasting—at the 5:2 version that is not dissimilar to what Jack Dorsey advocates. At the moment, much of the research is limited to animal studies, and research on humans is more challenging (so many more confounding factors!), but so far, the indicators are positive. Certainly, short of actual malnutrition or starvation, consistently reducing calories from the standard American overabundance can be good for your way of thinking in many ways.

Will it help improve my mood and outlook? "Mood" and "outlook" mean different things to different people, of course, and both—regardless of your personal definitions—are subject to influence from psychological and circumstantial factors that reach far beyond biology. However, your brain and body *do* have an influence on both, and so far the research into intermittent fasting as a positive influence on mood is encouraging, though not definitive.

One reality is that a serious commitment to intermittent fasting and/or OMAD will absolutely have an effect on your mood early on, as your body strives to adjust to this

THE JACK DORSEY WAY

entirely new lifestyle. For one thing, you're messing with your body's blood sugar, and spikes or drops in that physically affect brain function. Many people report increased irritability or a lack of focus—a kind of "brain fog" as they transition. You can hear frequent reports from other quarters, like the notorious "keto flu."

After the first few days, however, many people report a significant increase in energy and no "afternoon crash" that is so common for many of us. Combine that with the regularly reported improvement in sleep quality and duration, and—after that initial adjustment period—you might be able to look forward to a brighter, more positive outlook.

Will it help me control my blood sugar, blood pressure, and cholesterol? These are the claims you hear most often from a wide number of OMAD and intermittent fasting advocates. And since all of those conditions—especially diabetes—are very much influenced by diet, sleep, and physical activity, there are bound to be some effects on these numbers and risk levels if you get into OMAD. There have been a number of reliable studies that indicate that intermittent fasting does have a positive effect on blood sugar, but equally strong effects on blood pressure, insulin resistance, and inflammation weren't so clear.

But there are potential dangers here as well. If you have been diagnosed with type 2 diabetes, or even if you have been diagnosed as pre-diabetic, you *must* talk with your healthcare provider before you begin any kind of intermittent fasting program. Every case of type 2 diabetes is different;

some are more "sensitive" than others, depending on your personal biology and the state of progression of the disease. The good news is that intermittent fasting doesn't seem to trigger episodes of *low* blood sugar, known as hypoglycemia, but it might not help or may even hurt your blood sugar levels, especially dependent on what you eat when breaking your fast. So check first. And the same applies if you're already on medications for high blood pressure.

There's some small amount of evidence, still being investigated, that intermittent fasting can actually *increase* cholesterol levels, but that remains to be seen. Here again, let your healthcare providers know what you're doing, and monitor your "numbers" as you make the change and settle in to your new eating and activity patterns. You want everything to be pointed in a healthier direction.

Will it save me time? Once more, we're back to logic: Yes, it will. Think about how much time you spend on food and food-related activities every single day. Not just eating itself, of course, but the time spent on food preparation, food shopping, and even cleaning up. You'll be reducing that by huge amounts—maybe as much as 75 percent. And even if part of that time goes into longer, better sleep, you'll still be ahead of the game. This is one of the most frequently reported "unexpected consequences" of committing to intermittent fasting, and it's all good.

Will it save me money? Sure. It's really pure arithmetic. If you decrease the number of meals you eat by 70 percent, then you will decrease the money you spend by 70 percent.

We generally underestimate how much of our money we spend on food and food-related activities. And again, as with time: cookware and utility bills (after all, you'll be using significantly less water, natural gas, and/or electricity). You'll even be doing less laundry. Here, too, there are happy reports from OMAD advocates about the surprising financial impact OMAD has had on their lives.

Will it help me develop self-discipline? This is one of the benefits you see listed on OMAD websites and on videos all the time. It's hard to measure or even agree on, but two things seem certain: Committing to OMAD or intermittent fasting or both—in fact, committing to any of the tenets of the Jack Dorsey Way—gives you the *opportunity* to practice self-discipline. After all, you're making a promise to yourself to make some major changes in your life, and that requires some pretty significant restructuring. Second, in real terms, this relates to what we discussed above: *mindfulness.* "Self-discipline" is just a slightly more ominous term for the same thing, for *paying attention* and *commitment.*

Can you do it? *Will* you do it? OMAD and intermittent fasting don't so much *cause* an increase in self-discipline, but allows you to *practice* it.

Will it help me sleep better? Probably, at least a little. At one level, of course, you're reducing the level of fuel going into your body, so you will probably crave more sleep. You're also regulating the input of fuel, and therefore smoothing out your blood sugar levels—again, something that may encourage more and better sleep.

There's some evidence—and more research being done right now—that intermittent fasting can strengthen the power of your circadian rhythms (where things like work hours, late-night TV, and "time-shifting" fight against it in the modern world). As Michael J. Breus, a clinical psychologist who calls himself "The Sleep Doctor," has said, "A stronger, more synchronized circadian clock means an easier time falling asleep, staying asleep, and waking feeling refreshed on a regular basis. That combination of consistency and quality in a sleep routine is what we all want, to help us feel and function at our best, and to protect our health over time, and with age." He, and others, point to studies that show how intermittent fasting can help reduce disrupted sleep, but others show it may decrease REM sleep—which is the best kind for restfulness, tranquility, and healing.

All in all, intermittent fasting encourages structure in your life, and the idea of keeping open a twelve-hour period where you're not adding any fuel to the biological fire will almost certainly help your sleep quality and quantity, other physiological or psychological issues aside.

Will it help me live longer? This has to be the single most unmeasurable claim of all. For one thing, the population that has committed to a consistent OMAD or even intermittent fasting lifestyle in any form is still quite small and has only been present for a few years. It's virtually impossible to clinically validate if people who adopt and stick with OMAD will have a longer, much less healthier life.

That's not to say we don't have some hints. USC's National Institute on Aging and the Longevity Institute has been conducting animal studies on subjects that have been living an animal-appropriate version of intermittent fasting. Their findings indicate that, "In laboratory rats and mice, intermittent fasting has profound beneficial effects on many different indices of health and, importantly, can counteract disease processes and improve functional outcome in experimental models of a wide range of age-related disorders including diabetes, cardiovascular disease, cancers and neurological disorders such as Alzheimer's disease, Parkinson's disease and stroke." They propose that the cellular and molecular mechanisms triggered by intermittent fasting improve health and counteract disease processes... and also agree that further clinical trials are necessary to confirm and expand this conclusion.

It does stand to reason, however, if these practices improve your general health and help reduce or even eliminate age-related conditions like high blood pressure, high cholesterol, heart disease, and diabetes, then it's logical to assume you may actually live a longer, happier life. We can't prove it—yet—but it hasn't been disproven either.

Dangers, Will Robinson

Obviously, both OMAD and intermittent fasting are not a panacea, and there are risks involved—for anyone—taking on this commitment. They're not to be treated lightly.

Some groups of people should probably skip the OMAD/ Intermittent Fasting approach entirely. These groups include:

- People with type 1 diabetes or chronic low blood sugar (hypoglycemia). At the very least, they should consult with their endocrinologist or primary care provider first.
- People who have been diagnosed with type 2 diabetes, or even with prediabetes, should talk with their health-care providers before beginning.
- People with eating disorders like anorexia or bulimia, which can inadvertently encourage or reinforce their unhealthy conditions.
- People regularly taking medications that require food intake before dosage. (Some medications work more effectively with food, or food helps reduce gastrointes-tinal side effects. Others *require* the presence of food to work properly. Again: consult your healthcare provider.)
- Young people who are still actively growing (that is, children and adolescents, who need all the healthy food they can get).
- Women who are pregnant or breast-feeding.

Pay attention to Dr. Jason Fung, a nephrologist, bestselling author, and expert on intermittent fasting and low carb diets. His advice: *Be careful.* "You can be hungry," he said, "but you should not feel sick. If you do not feel well at any point, *you must stop.*" There is no shame in working with a physician before and during your transition to OMAD and intermittent fasting. Get all the help you can. After all, this isn't a short-term quick fix—this should be considered a long-term, even lifelong, transition, and you want to do it right.

No matter what benefits OMAD and intermittent fasting might offer, understand that the transition itself is going to be a shock to your system. During that transition period, especially in the first few days, you're likely to experience a range of effects, including, but not limited to:

- becoming extremely hungry
- shakiness, weakness, light-headedness, dizziness
- irritability
- inability to concentrate
- fatigue
- nausea
- blood pressure destabilization
- hypoglycemia (low blood sugar, even in those who do not have diabetes)
- dehydration

Even after the transition, there is substantial evidence that one of the most vulnerable times for your body is when you break your day-long or weekend-long fast, and your body rushes to accept and process the sudden influx of nourishment. You might even feel hungrier than you've felt in the past precisely because of this. This is why people with diagnosed and treatable eating disorders are on the "skip it" list. There is a very real increased risk of binge eating for people using OMAD or intermittent fasting, in those with the disorder and even in people who have never experienced this condition before.

Watch for it and respond swiftly and decisively with a visit to the right care provider.

And one more time: These health risks are real. They're not something that just *might* happen, or something you can dodge. Be honest about your current physical condition, your level of activity, the medications you're taking, and your plans for the future (like parenthood). Understand that this is a serious step you're taking—far more serious, in fact, than almost any other element in Jack Dorsey's plan. So be careful.

It should be noted that, according to a recent article from *Business Insider* early this year, Dorsey has extended his daily dinner regimen to weekends as well.

Is There a Better Fasting Alternative Than Jack Dorsey's Approach?

The field of intermittent fasting is wide and growing wider, and yes, there are a number of alternatives to Jack Dorsey's OMAD-plus-weekend fast approach.

As you begin your research, you'll see a lot of numbers. They usually describe the hours or days you're setting aside to eat (or not eat). There's "23:1", which is the numerical version of OMAD. There's "16:8," which restricts eating to just eight hours out of every twenty-four. And there's "5:2," which refers to days rather than hours: five days eating, two days fasting (Jack Dorsey's version is a particularly challenging hybrid of 23:1 and a two-day fast).

Some experts see more value in the 16:8 approach than the 23:1, but there is plenty of research yet to be done. Some proponents skip the numbering entirely and simply stop eating when it gets dark outside, then start again in the morning with breakfast.

Other options include **the 24-hour fast,** which generally lasts from dinner to dinner (or breakfast to breakfast). This might be a better option for people who need to take daily medications that benefit from or require food intake. It can also be much easier to incorporate into a "normal" work and life schedule for you and your family. There's also **the alternative daily fast**—one day on, one day off—where, generally speaking, you're allowed up to 500 calories on fasting days. If you do the math, you see it's slightly more intensive than the 5:2 approach, and may be either easier or more difficult to maintain over the long term, depending on your day-to-day (or every other day-to-day) lifestyle situation.

Interest and information on intermittent fasting is growing all the time. If any of these concepts interest you, look into it, and don't feel that Jack Dorsey's fairly aggressive approach to the concept is the only way you can...or the only one that will work for your particular set of circumstances and goals.

What to Expect, How to Succeed

Let's assume, for a moment, that you've decided to take the plunge. Be aware of one final reality: Most people who try OMAD or intermittent fasting, in almost any form, *don't* stick with it.

Honestly, it's hard. So much about modern life works against these kinds of major changes. But there are some things you can expect and prepare for, and some things you can do to increase the odds of long-term success.

First and foremost: *make a plan.* Do some honest self-appraisal and decide not only what your goals might be, but what version of OMAD and/or intermittent fasting will really, truly, work for you in the long run. And check out the box elsewhere in this chapter on "Choosing Your Window."

Remember, too, that you should not undertake OMAD or any version of intermittent fasting in a "bubble." Jack Dorsey's unique hybrid of 5:2 and fasting works for him because it is part of a larger commitment—to intense exercise and aerobic activity, to better sleep and rest, to better nourishment both physical and spiritual. Make OMAD and intermittent fasting part of *your* larger plan, too, not a substitute for it. It all has to work together.

Second: hope for the best, but prepare for the worst. Take a look again at that list of possible, temporary side-effects as you transition. Be sure to have a no-calorie beverage, whether it's water or unsweetened coffee or tea (if you've decided to include those beverages). Hydration is the issue here; you'd be surprised how much water you derive from eating food as opposed to drinking water, and you'll want to replace that water intake as you decrease your food consumption. By the same token, know how you're going to help with transition symptoms, from dizziness and irritability to "fasting headaches," so you're ready to respond to them.

Third: be sure to set goals—*incremental* goals, not just "I'm gonna do this forever!" Set a goal for the quality or quantity of food you consume when you're not fasting. And don't forget to congratulate yourself—*celebrate* yourself—when you reach those intermediate goals. They matter.

Fourth: track your progress. We'll talk more about this in the chapter on journaling, but nowhere will you find it more important than with OMAD and intermittent fasting, where there is a specific and relatively unforgiving structure. Don't rely on your memory or your good intentions; keep a log—on your phone, on the wall, or in a dedicated notepad with paper and pen. And keep track of the slip-ups as well as the successes. In the long run, you'll be glad to have that record of your progress that you can be proud of and learn from.

Finally: don't be afraid to reach out. Though this is something *you* have chosen to do, for yourself, don't hesitate to turn to family and friends for support as you embark on this journey. And there is a larger community available, too, both in your local geographic area and on the internet. Check our "resources" list at the end of the book for information on online forums; Google for local meet-ups for OMAD or fasting groups that meet regularly to supply exactly what you need.

Don't think it will be easy. It won't. But decide, even before you begin, if it's worth it. And if it is…it can happen.

How to Choose Your OMAD "Eating Window"

This may seem simple or straightforward at first, but think about it: *When* you decide to have your One Meal A Day is just as important as *what* you eat during that "window." It's a reflection of your entire day-to-day life and commitments, and if you're in this for the long haul, you'll want to optimize your chances of success by considering this part of the plan very carefully.

So sit down, take some time, and give it some thought. Here are just some of the things to consider:

What is your current, unchangeable schedule? What are your work hours? Do you have kids to get to school or meals that have to be prepared at a specific time? You don't want to put your "eating window" at a time when you simply won't be able to prepare and eat that one crucial meal of the day.

What is the current state of your health? Are you overweight or underweight? Do you have any chronic conditions, like diabetes, hypertension, or high cholesterol? Are you on any medications, and if so, when should you be taking them (and do they require or suggest food consumption immediately before or after you take them)? Be brutally honest here. Don't paint yourself a picture of where you'd *like* to be, but where you really are *now*. This will guide your decision on where to put your "eating window" and may inform your decision to proceed at all.

Do you have natural "up" or "down" times during the day? We all do. True, some of that "sleepy time" behavior is due to the food you eat and when you eat it, but we all have a natural set of biorhythms that also dictate when we're most awake and creative and when we're ready for a nap (or at least some downtime). Figure that timing out.

How are you going to deal with your hunger? And you *will* be hungry—it's inevitable. How do you think you'll react? Do you have a no-calorie beverage that will help? Do you have a friend or family member you can call? Would you benefit from some distracting activity that can help you for a few minutes, when things get tough? Don't assume that the hunger pangs won't really bother you. Instead, be ready to react in the best possible way when it comes calling.

What kind of support can you expect from friends or family? You've already talked to them about your plan. Now, how can they help? Are you someone who will benefit from a talk with a sympathetic friend or family member? Maybe it's best to go to the online forums or have a counselor or mentor on call who is ready and able to help. You don't have to do this alone, so don't try to.

What do you plan on eating when you break your fast? Think about that: You have one hour to eat in the standard OMAD configuration, but if you're planning on *cooking* what you eat, or preparing in it any way, you have to factor in that prep time as well. Are you doing it as part of a family's standard meal? Will you be on your own? How much time will that "best possible food" take to prepare (and include shopping and clean-up time in your calculations)?

How will you handle social interactions during your fast? If you have an active social life or a day that is structured, even in part, around family meals...consider it. If your "window" coincides with an all-important family meal, that's great...but it may not. Maybe it *can't*. But do you want (or would you prefer) to eat alone?

Okay...*now* you can pull out that day planner or notebook or tablet and decide on the best time of day for your meal. Now you can get serious about whether the weekend fast (or some other version of it) will work for you at all. Ask yourself the key question: *Is this something I want to be doing, CAN be doing in a year's time? In two years?* Remember you're thinking about a long-term lifestyle change here, not a quick fix. And as always: Test. Measure. Commit.

Why Fruit Juice is Bad for You (No, Really!)

You almost certainly don't want to hear this, and you will almost as certainly receive some blowback if you act on this new information, but here it is:

**Fruit juice—from concentrate, frozen, or fresh-squeezed—really isn't good for you.
You should eliminate or at least reduce
its use in your daily diet,
and it should not be part of your OMAD
or intermittent fasting food list.**

It's understandable—if entirely incorrect—to assume that orange juice is a health food. That's what we've been told for years. And after all, fruit juices are made from *fruits,* and we're constantly (and correctly) told that we should be *increasing* our intake of fruits and vegetables.

While it's true, the experts who are saying that are talking about *fresh, whole* fruits and vegetables, as close to their original form as possible (and we're not getting into the "cook vs raw" controversy—at least not here. Steaming, baking, and roasting your vegetables are fine. Have at it.).

But fruit juices, whether made by a machine or much more lovingly by you and your family, actually *reduce* the healthy aspects of the fruit and leave behind only two ingredients—one you can get far more easily, and One you don't really want: **water** and **sugar**.

Simply put: one or two pieces of *whole* fruit every day supply you with a wide range of vitamins, minerals, antioxidants, and fiber, along with a certain amount of sugar to make the medicine go down. There is almost nothing *not* good about that. But squeezing the juice out of eight to ten pieces of fruit, by any technology, *removes* most of the dietary fiber, some of the other trace elements that are part of that fiber, and concentrates all that sugar into a single serving.

In short: *That fruit juice you love so much contains just as much sugar and calories as a sugary soft drink...and sometimes even more.*

Why is one piece of fruit better than six or eight pieces squished together?

Lots of reasons, with "fiber" at the top of the list. Fiber has been proven, over and over, to lower cholesterol levels, to help control blood sugar, and to give you a healthier bowel. It helps you lose weight and is an essential part in a diet that helps you live longer. (Fun fact: The fiber you consume when you eat a whole orange actually emits a kind of "slime" that *slows down* the translation of that orange's sugar into the blood stream, reducing "spikes" in your blood sugar levels. That slime is missing from your glass of orange juice, even the kind with "pulp added.") Fruit also gives you chewing resistance, which is great for your teeth and digestion (ask any dentist if he prefers you eating one apple a day or drinking one big ol' glass of apple juice a day). Chewing resistance also means that the fructose in that fruit hits your liver more slowly— again, a good thing for your body.

What's more, fruit, as opposed to juice, is far more filling. Eating a single apple or orange satisfies you (look elsewhere in this chapter for a talk on *satiety*), and therefore the sugar intake is self-limiting. Yes, there's plenty of sugar in that fruit (for instance, your basic apple contains twenty-three grams of sugar, thirteen of which are fructose), but you're not going to sit down and eat seven or eight apples in a row—or even in a couple of days. So eating the complete fruit limits the shock that the sugar can cause to your liver, *and* you expose it to only a fraction of the amount of sugar to begin with.

Don't let the relatively small amounts of vitamins and minerals in a single piece of fruit fool you (you can and do get those from other sources every day). Instead, look at this:

A twelve ounce glass of Coca Cola contains 140 calories and forty grams (ten teaspoons!) of sugar.
A twelve ounce glass of apple juice contains <u>165</u> calories and <u>thirty-nine</u> grams of sugar.

It's for exactly this reason that endocrinologists and family practitioners tell their patients with newly diagnosed diabetes to take the orange juice off their breakfast table and out of the refrigerator. It's bad for them. And it's bad for you, your liver, and your weight control as well, whether you have diabetes or not.

This is true of virtually all fruit juices—orange, apple, and grape among them—even if no additional sugar is added. Obviously lemonade and other juices with added sugar fall into the same category.

This isn't to say, of course, that fruit juice is poison. You and your liver can stand an occasional small celebratory or polite glass, and you don't have to eliminate that lemonade from your Arnold Palmer. But downing six or eight ounces every morning as part of your "healthy breakfast" is not only unnecessary...it's doing damage to you. And because of their high caloric and low nutritive value, they shouldn't be a part of an OMAD or intermittent fasting menu at all.

The Harsh Reality of Weight Defense

Losing weight is one of the major reasons that people choose to commit to OMAD and intermittent fasting. They often do it in hopes that this strategy will help them lose more weight faster and keep it off longer.

The science to back up that notion is mixed at best, but the desire remains. And all too often—especially in highly structured commitments like One Meal a Day or intermittent fasting—a great deal of weight (so to speak) is put on the purely psychological issues of "willpower" or "self-discipline." This implies that success or failure in programs like OMAD is based solely, or at least over-whelmingly, on mental challenges. Mind over matter, as it were.

However, it's important to note that a number of recent studies point towards other, *biologically* based processes that have a huge influence on weight loss. One of these processes has become known as "weight defense."

Put simply: When a person loses as little as five to seven percent of their body weight, the body itself goes into panic mode. It thinks it has entered a time of famine, that nourishment is no longer easily available, so it begins to transmit specific hormones to the brain, changing thinking (and therefore behavior) in an attempt to increase food intake. In recent years, these changes in brain chemistry have been tracked and measured repeatedly, and their effects are clear. There are biochemical changes underway that are affecting:

- Hunger
- Satiety
- Perseverance

When weight defense kicks in, people find themselves hungrier than they've ever been...not because they are necessarily getting fewer calories or nutrients, but because the body wants *more* than the average, to make up for the perceived deficit. At the same time, the sense of satiety *decreases*, so even if calorie intake increases, the person suffering from weight defense does not feel full or satisfied; they have to actually eat more to feel as full as they're used to feeling. And finally, closing the loop, there is a marked increase in perseverance. Food becomes a top priority, almost an obsession. Thoughts of the next meal or any random food at all come to dominate thoughts of the present and the future.

These are not psychotically triggers; they are *biological*, and for the most part they are unavoidable. Obviously they differ in presence, timing, and severity according to the individual, but they are widely present in people attempting to lose weight, especially in those who are attempting to lose weight rapidly. And even more frustrating, your body doesn't care what your weight was when this began; you could be ten pounds or two hundred pounds above your goal weight, and the weight defense mechanism will still kick in when you rapidly lose more than about seven percent of your body weight.

The result is what is often called "plateauing"—a sudden decrease in weight loss after a steep, fast down-curve. You may or may not gain back some of the weight you've lost, but almost certainly your rate of decrease will slow or even stop for a while, at least until your body is convinced you are no longer starving and decreases those signaling chemicals.

How long will the "plateau" last? Once again, it depends on the individual. It can be anything from a few days to a few weeks, but eventually the obsession with the food and the sense of hunger will ease.

The best you can do in these situations is to know that it is not just your "willpower," or some psychological "flaw" that is keeping you from losing more weight as rapidly as you like. This is, in fact, a result of a biochemical defense mechanism, not some character flaw. Don't lose heart or commitment. Stick to the plan and do your best to be patient… and know that eventually—though not soon enough!—the weight defensive mechanism will dissipate and your weight loss will continue.

What Foods to Eat? What Things to Drink?

One of the most commonly asked questions of OMAD advocates and enthusiasts is, *what should I eat during my one hour a day?* As with so many other aspects of this ever-growing and changing movement, the answers you'll hear to that question are many and wildly varied. Some "experts" will suggest you eat anything you like, and as much of it as you can stand—whatever you crave. Others—like Jack Dorsey—suggest sticking to healthy, nutrient-rich foods in generous amounts—fruits, vegetables, whole grains, and lean proteins. It's probably a good idea for you to decide in which camp you're going to pitch your tent as you complete your OMAD plan, but know that wherever you land, you won't be alone.

One thing virtually everyone agrees on: drink water. Most people derive most of the water they consume every day not from beverages, but as part of the food they eat, so if your food volume is decreasing by as much as two-thirds, you'll want to counter that with plenty of water all day long.

Can that include other zero-calorie beverages, like coffee or tea? Here again, experts are split. Most seem to allow for unsweetened coffee and tea, but others point out that coffee and tea may contain xenobiotics that put a burden on your liver and should be avoided.

You may want to increase your salt intake as well. Unlike sugar, your body actually needs a certain amount of salt every day to do its job, and it derives most of that from dietary salt, not from the added sprinkles on your snacks. If you are decreasing your food-mass by 75 percent or so, you may want to consider salt tablets or other supplements to make sure you're giving your body what it needs.

Finally, strongly consider a food diary. We've mentioned this elsewhere in this chapter, and we will talk about the benefits of journaling in general in our last chapter, but here especially: Knowing how many calories, and maybe even how many grams of fat, carbohydrates, and proteins you've taken in during your single meal a day can be of great help at gauging your overall health. It's easy to do, whether you use electronic tools or pen-and-paper, but don't rely just on your memory or good intentions. Record the facts and refer to your performance later, as part of an ongoing commitment to self-improvement.

USING A STANDING DESK

**Dorsey has a standing desk
in his home office.**

J ack Dorsey almost off-handedly mentions that he uses a standing desk at work, but it's actually an important aspect of his life and an equally valuable innovation for most people working in the modern world.

Standing desks are one response to a staggering new threat to twenty-first century health: what is commonly referred to as *the sedentary lifestyle.* Let's talk a bit about it, the scientifically validated damage it's already doing, and what we can do about it. *Then* we'll talk about standing desks.

"The Standing Disease"

News flash: the world has changed. Truly, we often don't realize how much it's changed…or how those changes have changed *us.*

Barely fifty years ago, a huge chunk of American ingenuity and enterprise was focused on the creation of "labor-saving devices"—bits of technology that would make it easier for men and women to get through the day. From the perspective of the third decade of the twenty-first century, it's actually hard to imagine what day-to-day life was like immediately after the Second World War. Though most of America was enjoying indoor plumbing and electrical wiring (in many cases for the first time in history), the rest of life was still very time-consuming and exhausting. Everything from the gathering and preparing of food to simple transportation to and from work required significant physical effort. Even technology like electric mixers or flat irons, much less typewriters, were in short supply, and devices we now think of as commonplace, like personal computers, televisions of all shapes and sizes, and smart phones were decades away from invention.

Beginning in the 1960s—a little more than half a century ago—all that began to change. Here are just a few of the statistics:

- According to the American Heart Association, sedentary jobs have increased 83 percent since 1950.
- In 1970, only two in ten working Americans were in jobs that required only light activity (basically sitting at a desk), while three in ten were in jobs requiring high-energy output (construction, manufacturing, farming). By 2000—just thirty years later—more than four in ten adults were in light-activity jobs, whereas two in ten were in high-activity jobs. That's a doubling of desk jobs and a one-third decrease in physical jobs, in essentially a single generation.

- In 2003, nearly six in ten working adults used a computer on the job and more than nine in ten children used computers in school.
- Between 1989 and 2009, the number of households with a computer and internet access increased from 15 percent to 69 percent. Almost a *400 percent* increase in twenty years.
- The average American watches four hours of television a day and spends an average of one hour a day in a car. Both of those are all-time highs.

This is more than just a grumble about the "good old days." These massive changes in social behavior have resulted in equally massive changes in our collective health. In a recent article for Johns Hopkins, Dr. Erin Michos, Associate Director of Preventive Cardiology at the Ciccarone Center for the Prevention of Heart Disease, talked at length about exactly how all this sedentary behavior has hurt us.

Back in 2015, in the *Annals of Internal Medicine*, Michos commented on a wide range of studies and found that people sitting for long periods of time had higher incidences of heart disease, type 2 diabetes, and cancer. Quite simple, he said, "Sedentary behavior can increase your risk of dying, either from heart disease or other medical problems."

Not surprisingly, the sedentary lifestyle becomes an even bigger issue the older we get. One recent estimate from the Department of Health and Human Services indicate that fully two-thirds of older adults sit for more than eight hours a day, while less than a third could be considered physically active.

It's true that committing to thirty minutes of physical activity a day—like Jack Dorsey recommends in his walking and HIIT activity—helps counteract some of that damage. But research shows pretty definitively that all that sitting *does* blunt the effects of moderate physical activity. High levels of exercise can help, Dr. Michos said, but, "even for people with high levels of activity, there seems to be a threshold around ten hours of sitting. Research shows that if you sit more than ten hours, your cardiovascular risk really goes up." It seems that prolonged sitting, whether you're at the computer or watching television, can increase your chance of developing potentially fatal blood clots in the deep veins of the legs (the technical term is "venous thrombosis")—maybe increase the risk by *70 percent*, compared to people who never watch TV.

From an evolutionary standpoint, this makes perfect sense. The human body, after all, was designed to *move*, not to sit in once place. It's a survival characteristic. And we have only recently shifted from an "active" to a "sedentary" species—recently as in the last fifty years after 20,000 or more years on the planet.

And it's not as if "not getting exercise" and "sitting around" are the same thing. In fact, the latter is significantly more harmful than the former. Look at it this way:

- *Sedentary behavior* is defined as sitting or lying down, and expending very little energy.
- *Light-intensity activity* is defined as standing, slow walking, basically *moving around*.

And the difference is important because it's so widespread. Basically, **one in four US adults spend about 70 percent of their waking hours sitting, 30 percent in light activities, and little or no time in exercise.**

Both sedentary and light-intensity activities are distinct from the kind of exercise that Jack Dorsey and his colleagues perform when they walk to work or perform HIIT. And with new technologies like the accelerometer, researchers are actually able to see the different effects that sitting has, compared to simple moving around. Among other negative effects, sitters are showing:

- An increase in central adiposity (that's belly fat to you and me—a larger waist circumference)
- Higher triglyceride levels (that's cholesterol)
- Increased insulin resistance (a major factor in diabetes)
- Increased cardiovascular disease
- Increase all-cause mortality (or, to put it bluntly, a greater chance of dying for any health-related reason)

All this research makes one thing abundantly, even painfully, clear: Most people working in today's world face the dual challenge of too little exercise *and* too much sitting.

How to Counter the Sedentary Lifestyle and the Damage It Does

Evelyn O'Neill, manager of outpatient exercise programs at the Harvard-affiliated Hebrew Rehabilitation Center, recently told a Harvard University publication that, "Sitting is the new smoking, in terms of health risks. Lack of movement is perhaps more to blame than anything for a host of health problems." And the American Academy of Pediatrics has been telling parents for years that they should limit their children's screen time to no more than a couple of hours per day. The fact of the matter is that they should be telling themselves and their adult friends and family members exactly the same thing. *Everyone* needs to get out of their chairs more often, at work and at home.

The good it would do would be immediately apparent and extensive. Experts tell us that every minute of sedentary behavior that is replaced with light activity—not even "real" exercise, just *light activity*—would expend one additional kilocalorie. It's not much, but it's significant…and it builds up.

All you really have to do is *move around instead of sitting all day*. It's really no more challenging than that. Simply standing more can help you lose weight and keep it off (according to a review published in the *European Journal of Preventive Cardiology*). Everyday activities that incorporate more walking can build up your leg muscles, too, which may help you live longer. Researchers have found that loss of leg muscle strength and mass is associated with slower walking speeds among older adults, and slower speeds are linked to a lower ten-year survival rate for people after the age of seventy-five.

How can you make this happen? Do what Dr. Michos does: **"I make an effort to get up and move around every hour.** I try to find as many excuses as possible to walk throughout the day. I'll ask myself: Do I really have to send that email to my colleague down the hall, or can I just walk over to her office?"

Most experts agree that as little as thirty minutes of light activity, as little as three days a week, will effectively counter most of the long-term effects of sedentary behavior—on top of your other more demanding exercise. So aim for that. And keep in mind that you don't have to do it all at once. Plenty of research indicates that you can break it up in very small increments, as little as ten minutes at a time, and still derive most of the health benefits from it.

Here's a simple rule of thumb: For every twenty minutes of sitting, try to stand for eight minutes and move around for two minutes. Evelyn O'Neill was recently quoted in a Harvard health publication: "Even if you aren't sweating or feeling like you're working hard, you are still moving your arms and legs, stimulating your muscles, and working your joints."

Here are just a few ideas:

- Get in the habit of staging (and encouraging others to stage) walking meetings instead of sit-down meetings.
- Every two hours, get up and walk for at least five minutes..
- Practice heel raises by standing up and rising on your toes. "Try it while you brush your teeth or make breakfast," says O'Neill.
- If you find yourself on the phone, walk around or stand until the call is completed.
- Use reference books or canned goods as dumbbells, at work or at home, and aim for ten to twenty biceps curls.
- Practice "stand-and-sit exercises," rising from a chair without using your arms and then sitting back down again. Ten reps would be great.

Bottom line: "There's a lot you can do to be more active," Dr. O'Neill reminds us. "Exercise doesn't always have to be intense to be effective, and there are many opportunities in your daily life to sneak in extra movement. You just need to do it."

And then, of course, there's the standing desk…

How to Choose a Standing Desk

Call them what you want: standing desks, stand-up desks, sit-stand desks, sit-to-stand desks—it doesn't matter. What's important is to find one that works for you, so that you don't join the gathering throng of people (like those who buy exercise bikes, treadmills, and free weights) who use them for a couple of weeks and then set it low and drag in a chair. So here are some steps to go through.

Step One: What exactly is it you do?

Standing desks come in two flavors: those that can be adjusted for sitting *or* standing work, and those that are designed for standing only. Think about what it is you do all day long, and whether some of that work really is better performed while sitting. If you really do plan on standing part of the time and sitting part of the time, go for the adjustable designs.

Step Two: Are you going for a whole new desk or an add-on?

You aren't required to throw out your old favorite piece of furniture just to get healthy. There may very well be add-on options available. Getting a desk-top adjustable unit may be possible, but it won't be any cheaper than a full, new desk, and you can spend a lot of time trying to find that perfect fit for your existing arrangement, but again: Be honest. Which way do you want to go?

Step Three: How adjustable should it be?

Short answer: as adjustable as you can get, given the space you have to fill, the surface space you require (depth *and* width), how heavy-duty it needs to be to accommodate what it has to carry (computers, speakers or other equipment, shelving, and so on.), and your own personal needs and preferences.

Take a few minutes to measure the exact "comfort height" you're after. Try this:

1. Sit comfortably at your current desk, in your current chair. Put your feet flat on the floor, and pretend to type or draw or handwrite—whatever you do most of the time.

2. Now measure the distance from the floor to the underside of your outstretched elbow. That measurement is roughly the height your keyboard should be in your new desk.

3. Now stand up and take the same measurement, pantomiming where you would want that keyboard or desk surface to be if you were standing.

4. So now you know the minimum and maximum levels of adjustability for your future standing desk—

one that you'll be happy to use at both extremes and everything in between.

Step Four: What other accessories, accommodations, or bits of hardware might you want?

Be sure to give full thought to the real-world application of your standing desk and ask yourself what other additional pieces of hardware would help you get your job done. For instance:

- Do you want to opt for an electric or pneumatic adjustment, or are you fine with a crank?
- Do you want an adjustable monitor arm to accommodate movement and convenience (this is particularly helpful if you collaborate or do presentations from your desk)?
- Do you want or need a keyboard tray that can be adjusted to go lower than the desk surface (and why you would need that if the desk itself is adjustable)?
- Do you want a footrest?
- Would you benefit from a padded anti-fatigue mat under your feet? If you anticipate spending much of your workday on your feet, pads are highly recommended.

Step Five: Get some recommendations and advice.

There are enough standing desk users out there now that it shouldn't be too difficult to find someone—maybe even in your own office, in your family, or among your professional colleagues—who has been using one for a while now. Find that person (or more than one!) and ask them how they like it, what they should have thought of before they bought it, and ask for any advice they might have about making the change. They might even have some brand recommendations—or wave-offs—when it comes to models or manufacturers. It's well worth the time.

Finally: Don't forget a chair.

Yes, you still need one. But maybe you don't need that costly ergonomic number that you used before; hopefully you'll be spending far less time in it than you have in the past. You might even want to consider an adjustable stool, with or without a back...and look on the bright side: if it becomes uncomfortable after an hour or so, that can serve as a reminder that it's time to get up and move around. That light activity is still the goal....

Expect an adjustment period.

Do yourself a favor: As excited as you might be about your new desk, don't try standing in front of it for a whole shift on your first day. You'll hurt yourself. Instead, try to alternate standing and sitting every thirty to sixty minutes. But do keep rough track of how much time you're actually standing in that first week. And the second. And a month later when the honeymoon is over and the "new desk smell" has faded away. There are actual, demonstrable health benefits to integrating a standing desk into your life. Don't shrug it off.

Though the use of a standing desk may be one of the smallest and least "radical" things that Jack Dorsey includes in his regimen, this decision can have major positive effects on your day-to-day life and your long-term health.

Give it some thought, and go do some shopping.

NEAR-INFRARED LIGHT

**When Jack Dorsey is working at the standing
desk in his home office, he also uses a lamp
with a single near-infrared bulb.**

J ack Dorsey hasn't discussed his use of near-infrared radiation (NIR) light very much, but let's take this opportunity to talk about the health benefits of NIR and its cousins Red Light Therapy and Low Level Light Therapy, (LLLT) in general…if there are any.

Like many other alternative healthcare strategies, light therapy in general and NIR in particular are subject to many wild claims in benefits, and often cite "scientific studies" to back up those claims; but when you get down to the details, real evidence is spotty and best and non-existent at worst. That is not to say that light therapy is useless or a sham; it just means there are not large and well-constructed studies that affirm its benefits. If you decide to include it in your healthcare regimen, it's something you would largely have to take on faith rather than science.

The popularity and inherent credibility of light-based therapy is entirely understandable; it's something humans have believed as far back as history can trace. Even the ancient Egyptians practiced *heliotherapy*, or healing through the use of the sun's rays, some 3,500 years ago.

It's also true that more than half of the energy transmitted by the sun is near-infrared radiation, and modern-day electric lighting contains almost no near-infrared radiation. Today, you receive hundreds of times more NIR when you're outside than when you're inside. But does this lack of exposure actually have any negative effect on your health? And does "amping up" the amount of NIR you receive, through incandescent bulbs of light-emitting diodes (LEDs) really do you any good?

The fact is nobody knows.

If you were to do any research on light therapy, you would find yourself tumbling down a cyber-rabbit hole filled with numbers, formulae, and acronyms. LLLT alone is also known as "low level laser therapy," "cold laser therapy," "laser biostimulation," and most often "photobiomodulation."

Amongst all the jargon, however, one thing is worth noting: There is a difference between "red light therapy" and "near infrared therapy," based on the wavelengths that are used. One easy distinction is that red light therapy involves visible light; NIR involves infrared light from beyond the visual spectrum. Another important distinction is that red light therapy affects the surface of the human skin, while the wavelengths associated with NIR actually penetrate human flesh, and—in theory, anyway—affect the cells *under* the surface. How much they affect them, and in what way, is open to controversy, even after years of study.

Beyond that, making any generalizations about the need for or therapeutic values of any version of light therapy is very difficult. This is due, in part, to the confounding factors of *irradiance* (that is, the level of radiation received) and *dosage* (that is, the way in which that radiation is transmitted). It's even more confusing when you consider that human tissue has an annoying tendency to react differently to exactly the same amount of radiation if it's received in a pulse as opposed to over a long period of time. Even comparing the effects of man-made light generated by any technology to the near-infrared radiation you receive when you're outside is problematic, since that "natural" exposure can vary wildly depending on the intensity of the sun, the amount of moisture in the air, even the geography of any given exposure. In short, it's damn near impossible to draw any general conclusions, or make any valid general statements, about the value of light therapy for humans, no matter what the company websites say.

The (Speculative) Benefits of NIR

Various experts—many of them associated with manufacturers and distributors of light therapy products—have a long list of potential benefits from near-infrared therapy. Among the claims:

- Reduction in body fat
- Greater production of white blood cells
- Improved circulation

- Wound healing
- Skin rejuvenation
- Improved flexibility
- Reduction in inflammation
- Increase in energy
- Relief of muscle and joint pain
- Anti-aging benefits
- Increased collagen production
- Treatment of depression and Seasonal Affect Disorder (SAD)
- Hair restoration or the slowing or end of hair loss
- Treatment of autoimmune and hormone-related conditions
- Improved cognitive function
- Increased strength, endurance, and muscle mass

That's quite a list, and many of the effects listed here are essentially immeasurable. What's true of almost all of them is though there have been many, *many* studies relating to Low Level Light Therapy, Red Light Therapy, and Near Infrared Radiation, virtually all of the studies have been quite small and short-term, many have been inconclusive, and many were sponsored by companies that make therapeutic products or otherwise profit from light therapy. That calls the results of almost all of them into question in any number of ways.

Nonetheless, the proponents of light therapy in all its forms love to claim that it has been scientifically "proven" to be effective. Here are a couple of "back-up" assertions you're likely to come across if you do any reading:

- **"NASA research has found that the NIR electromagnetic frequency band of energy penetrates deeply into the body and can have a healing effect on our individual cells."** It's true that a branch of the National Aeronautics and Space Administration conducted tests on using NIR in wound healing and cell regeneration in the early 1980s and found that NIR does exactly that, but apparently that research has never been duplicated, and even then it was performed under very strict guidelines—that stuff about "irradiance and dosage" comes into play again—so it isn't really fair to extrapolate those findings into validation of the entire field.

- **"A wide range of studies shows that...[followed by one of more of the claims listed above]."** The problem here is that many of those studies apply to LLLT. And as an excellent piece from the Illuminating Engineering Society points out, the term "Low Level" can be misleading. Many of these studies focused on the use of high-power medical lasers used for tissue removal, cutting, and cauterization, so applying those finding, however valid or invalid, to Red Light Therapy or NIR really isn't appropriate.

So Is NIR Safe?

Probably. Again, there is little definitive research, but given what we've got, there is very little evidence that exposure to near-infrared radiation, from LEDs or incandescent lights alike, will do you any harm. There has been some research in the last decade that suggests possible aging of the skin and even skin cancer, but here again, it's inconclusive.

The single greatest risk to a consumer has more to do with your bank balance than biology. Many of the red light and NIR devices—bulbs, lamps, irradiators, and even wrapping blankets for weight reduction—can be very expensive and may do very little good.

Is NIR Effective?

The results are mixed. Here are just a few of the nuggets you'll find if you do a deep dive into NIR research:

- NIR does seem to activate anti-inflammatory processes and is widely used in veterinary medicine to treat sprains and bone fractures, as well as to speed the healing of wounds.
- The ability of NIR to induce weight reduction has been studied extensively, but there is no evidence that it does.
- NIR seems to have a beneficial effect on collagen and elastin production, though the precise biological mechanism at work is unclear. Skin treatment with infrared radiation may be effective and safe, and it may also be useful in the treatment of photo-aged skin.

- There have been some promising studies for using NIR in treating traumatic brain injury, though three randomized, placebo-controlled clinical trials for the treatment of stroke yielded mixed results.

- Those brain injury studies did show, in some cases, that symptoms such as headache, insomnia, irritability, anxiety, depression, suicidal ideation, fatigue, and memory or concentration difficulties were resolved or greatly reduced and did not recur.

The bottom line is that we just don't know...yet. Much larger animal and human studies are needed. And until there is valid and verifiable scientific study, there's no guarantee that investing your time and money on NIR equipment or light therapy will yield the kind of results you're looking for.

However...

Now is as good a time as any to bring up a touchy subject: **The placebo effect.**

Make no mistake: This isn't a condescending dismissal, a "nice" way to say, "It's all in your head," or "If it feels good, do it." The fact is that the placebo effect is a very real, very measurable phenomenon that affects a far larger proportion of adults than previously thought, and a great deal of research into this amazing mind/body interaction has taken place in recent years. In fact, many healthcare providers now believe that, under the right circumstances, a placebo can be just as effective as traditional treatments.

In a recent piece from Harvard University, Professor Ted Kaptchuk of Harvard-affiliated Beth Israel Deaconess Medical Center said, "The placebo effect is more than positive thinking.... It's about creating a stronger connection between the brain and body and how they work together." And it's important to realize that placebos are not *replacements* for traditional procedures. Tales of miracle cures and overnight remissions aside, placebos work best when dealing with *symptoms* of disease. "Placebos may make you feel better, but they will not cure you," says Kaptchuk. "They have been shown to be most effective for conditions like pain management, stress-related insomnia, and cancer treatment side effects like fatigue and nausea."

How is this even possible? The research into understanding this complex neurological process is ongoing. Some experts believe it's from an increase in "feel-good" neurotransmitters like dopamine or endorphins; others attribute it to the production of an enzyme called COMT. The list of challenges that respond best to placeboes continues to grow. They include:

- Anxiety and depression
- Back pain
- Chemotherapy-related illness
- Migraine headaches
- Post-operative pain
- Post-traumatic stress disorder

Now take another look at that list of the ailments and complaints that NIR was supposed to address...and notice how many of them are related to *symptoms* rather than *causes*.

Food for thought.

And here's the craziest thing of all:

**The Placebo Effect works even when you
know you're getting a placebo.**

Until quite recently, scientists thought that triggering the placebo effect was based on deception. If you let the patient know that they were getting a sugar pill, or being treated with an ineffective procedure, the effect itself will disappear or at least be blunted.

But in 2014, a study published in *Science Translational Medicine* took two groups of people suffering from migraines. One received an actual migraine drug, labeled as such. The other received a placebo labeled "Placebo." And the researchers found that the placebo was *50 percent as effective* as the actual medication...even when the subjects *knew* it was a placebo.

Scientists measured this by testing how people reacted to migraine pain medication. One group took a migraine drug labeled with the drug's name, another took a placebo labeled "placebo," and a third group took nothing. The researchers discovered that the placebo was 50 percent as effective as the real drug to reduce pain after a migraine attack.

Similar experiments by other researchers saw similar results with people who were dealing with irritable bowel syndrome. And elsewhere with back pain and hay fever. There are even startling and promising results with placebos and Parkinson's Disease.

As research into the placebo effect continues, it becomes even more fascinating. Some inquiries indicate that the branding and color of the placebo pill can have an effect on patients; it may be true that people who score higher on tests that measure "optimism" and "friendliness" do better with placebos; there is some evidence placebos can increase creative and cognitive performance. And some studies indicate that the percentage of people who are susceptible to placebo effects has been growing in recent decades.

The point is that *believing* in something, having *hope,* and a willingness to try new things has a real and measurable effect. And as long as it's not doing you any damage, and as long as you're not forgoing proven effective treatments and substitute a placebo in its place, why not try it? Whether it's Near Infrared Radiation, Meditation, and kale…at least part of your long-term health *is* in your head. And that's exactly where it should be.

TAKING DAILY VITAMIN AND MINERAL SUPPLEMENTS

"The only supplements I take are daily multivitamins and vitamin C, a lot of vitamin C," Jack Dorsey says.

J ack Dorsey believes in vitamin supplements…and so does almost everyone else in the United States. Some experts measure the percentage of Americans who take daily multivitamins at more than 70 percent, and with an even higher percentage among seniors.

Would you then believe that you don't really need them at all? Ask almost any nutritionist, dietitian, or healthcare professional and they'll tell you that if you eat a decent diet, you'll get all the vitamins you need on a daily basis (and the sad fact is, you'll probably get most of them, most of the time, even if you *don't* eat a diet that's all that healthy). Basic nutrition in this modern world is ridiculously easy to find, even when you're not looking for it. Vitamins and minerals are all over the place. Pills are not required. They're not only expensive; in some cases they can actually make your health worse, or even put you in danger.

Just as many of us have a deeply embedded mistrust of the medical establishment and Big Pharma, we have an almost-as-powerful deeply embedded *trust* in a wide range of alternative or preventive measures that really don't work at all. And through a fortunate—for them—"guilt by association," we trust many of the companies that create these bogus alternatives, often far more than they deserve.

Americans spend more than $30 billion dollars on vitamin and mineral supplements each year. That's more than one hundred dollars for every man, woman, and child in the country. And the companies that manufacture, market, and distribute those supplements know exactly what they're doing…and what they're doing is very little to help you live a healthier life.

A decades-long string of research projects, reports, and trials confirm their complete ineffectiveness. A recent article in the *New York Times* said it very succinctly: "A multivitamin/mineral supplement contains none of the fiber in fruits and vegetables, and to provide the amount of daily calcium recommended (1,000 milligrams for adults, rising to 1,200 for women over 50 and men over 70), the combination pill would be too big for most people to swallow."

So why do we keep buying them? Because of the deeply ingrained American desire for The Magic Pill, the one painless medication with no side effects that will keep us healthy and let us live forever. It's so much easier to search for (or blithely accept) its existence than to deal with the more demanding reality: The only real secret to health and a long life is to eat well, get regular exercise, get plenty of sleep, and don't smoke or drink alcohol to excess. That really will do the trick. And so far, nothing else gets you to that goal nearly as well.

That's not to say that vitamin supplements are all bad. They're absolutely necessary for some specific subgroups, and a few research papers have found possible risk reductions for stroke or cancer after prolonged use. But these outcomes are lonely voices in a sea of data that confirms the opposite conclusion. As Dr. JoAnn Manson, a professor of medicine at Harvard Medical School says, "Supplements are never a substitute for a balanced, healthful diet, and they can be a distraction from healthy lifestyle practices that convey much greater benefits."

And let's bear in mind too that *vitamins are not regulated by the Food and Drug Administration* the way that prescription medications and almost every food sold in a grocery store are. The supplement manufacturers can make any claims they want, and they can put whatever they want in those tablets, capsules, and elixirs without an accurate list of the ingredients on the label. The sad fact is you know more about what goes into a box of cake mix than you do about your multivitamin, and at least you can be sure the cake mix is free of contaminants, and that you're getting the same cake mix in every box you buy. That's not a solid bet when it comes to supplements.

So if not vitamin supplements...then what?

It's actually pretty simple: *Eat the right foods.* Let's go through a list of all the vitamins and minerals that nutritional scientists know we need—after years of research and advice that have resulted in Americans living longer and healthier lives than any generation before them. What you'll probably find is that you're already well—or at least well *enough*—already, or that small adjustments in your eating patterns—even if you're moving into OMAD or some other restricted eating pattern—will give you everything you need and more without the involvement of any magic pills.

Let's begin with the quintessentially popular vitamin that Jack Dorsey mentioned and everyone knows, then work our way down the rest of the list…

Vitamin C

Vitamin C, aka ascorbic acid, helps your body form blood vessels, cartilage, muscle, and collagen in bones. Vitamin C is also vital to your body's healing process and does wonderful things for your immune system. It even helps reduce your risk of chronic diseases. It's a major player.

However, it's not a miracle drug. Over the years, Vitamin C has been given credit for a great many things that it really doesn't deserve. Among them:

- There's no solid evidence that Vitamin C prevents cancer. Eating a diet rich in fruits and vegetables might, but not an oral Vitamin C supplement in any dosage or frequency.
- Taking a Vitamin C supplement won't prevent the common cold. There's some evidence that people who take Vitamin C regularly might have the cold for a few days less, but there are a host of confounding factors

(each person's overall diet and health, level of self-care, and even the placebo effect) that calls even that minor advantage into question.

Since our body doesn't make any Vitamin C on its own, you have to bring it on board regularly. So concentrate on including foods high in Vitamin C in your diet every day. These include oranges, red and green peppers, strawberries, black currants, broccoli, brussels sprouts, and even potatoes—yes, potatoes.

Finally, don't think that adding an oral supplement on top of good eating will increase your protection. Sadly, it doesn't work that way. Oral Vitamin C supplements *can* have side effects, especially if you're taking mega-doses. All your favorites: nausea, vomiting, heartburn, cramps, insomnia, headaches—even an elevated risk of kidney stones. And it doesn't work and play well with other substance like medications with aluminum, chemotherapy drugs, estrogen, statins, and even Warfarin, Coumadin, and Juvonen, to name a few.

Vitamin B1

Vitamin B1, aka thiamin, helps to break down and release energy from the food you eat and keeps your nervous system healthy. You can get plenty from peas, fresh and dried fruit, eggs, liver, and so much more. Like Vitamin C and others, your body can't make it or store it, so you need to have it in your food every day. In this case, there don't seem to be any side effects from taking too much thiamin, but why tempt fate?

Vitamin B2

Vitamin B2, aka riboflavin, keeps your skin, eyes, and nervous system healthy; and like its buddy thiamin, it aids in the release of energy in food. You'll find it in dairy products like milk and eggs and even rice. By the way, UV light destroys riboflavin, so keep your rice and eggs—and obviously your milk!—out of direct sunlight. Thankfully, there's no known side effects from taking too much thiamin (that is, more than forty milligrams a day, which you can easily get from a healthy diet).

Vitamin B3

Vitamin B3 also goes by the name of niacin, and it works with its brothers and sisters to release energy and keep your nervous system and skin healthy. You'll find it in abundance in meat, fish, dairy, and wheat flour. And you need it every day. High doses of nicotinic acid—one of the two kinds of niacin—can cause your skin to flush, and overdosing over a long period of time could lead to liver damage.

Pantothenic acid

You probably haven't heard of pantothenic acid, since it doesn't have a fancy Number-Letter name like its buddies. But it works with many of the other vitamins and minerals to aid in digestion and energy transmission, and you'll find it in almost all meats and vegetables, especially potatoes, tomatoes, broccoli, and whole grains. And yes, you need it every day. There are no known side effects from overdose, but no confirmed benefits from megadoses, either.

Vitamin B6

Vitamin B6, aka pyridoxine, is especially good at breaking down protein and carbohydrates. It also helps form red blood cells, and we all need those. You'll find it in pork, poultry, chicken, fish, peanuts, potatoes, soy beans, and so much more. And be careful: Overdosing on B6 can lead to a loss of feeling in arms and legs—a little gem knows as *peripheral neuropathy*—and if you take large amounts for long enough, that effect can be permanent.

Vitamin B7

Vitamin B7, or biotin, helps the body break down fat. This is an interesting one: The bacteria that naturally live in your bowel make biotin on their own, so it's not clear that you need to bring more on board at all. It's present in many foods you should be eating anyway, but in small amounts (which you may not need in any event).

Vitamin B9

Vitamin B9 often goes by its popular alias, folate, or its manmade cousin, folic acid. It's another vitamin that helps form red blood cells and has great positive effects in the development of healthy babies (that's why mothers are often told to take folic acid supplements). You'll find it in leafy green vegetables, cruciform veggies like broccoli, even brussels sprouts and peas. Your body can't store it long-term, so you need to ingest it fairly frequently. Though too much folic acid doesn't directly harm you, it can effectively mask the symptoms of another vitamin deficiency—B12—which can do real damage if it's not detected and treated. This is especially common in older people, since we often lose the ability to absorb Vitamin B12 as we get older.

Vitamin B12

Vitamin B12 makes red blood cells, and a lack of it could lead to a serious condition called *B12 deficiency anemia*. Meat, salmon, and dairy products all have Vitamin B12, but it generally isn't found in great quantities in plant-based foods, so strict vegetarians and vegans may not be getting enough. This is one of the rare instances where an oral supplement may be necessary for some people.

Vitamin A

Vitamin A, aka retinol, is almost as powerful as Vitamin C. It's a big help to your immune system; it helps keep your skin healthy, and it even helps with night vision. You'll find it in eggs and cheese and oily fish. Liver and pate are especially rich in vitamin A—so rich, in fact, that you can risk having too much on board if you eat liver more than once a week (which is why it is not recommended for pregnant women). Another fun fact: Your body converts beta-carotene into Vitamin A, and you can find that in yellow, red, and green leafy plants, and yellow fruit like mangos, papayas, and apricots. And Vitamin A from any source can be stored for future use, so you don't need to ingest it every day. Too much Vitamin A—which is, ironically, easy to absorb if you're taking supplements that include A, or enjoy too much of certain foods—may lead to osteoporosis and weaker bones. It's one of the great reasons *not* to take supplements.

Vitamin E

Vitamin E helps keep your skin and eyes healthy and is a great aid to the immune system. Plant oils like corn and olive oil have it, as do nuts and seeds and wheat germ. And this particular vitamin *is* stored for future use, so you don't need to eat it every day. There is a possibility that too much Vitamin E could lead to strokes, causing bleeding in the brain, but that research is continuing. Beyond that, there are no generally agreed-upon side effects for overconsumption.

Vitamin K

Vitamin K is essential for blood clotting and wound healing and probably helps keep bones healthy. Go to your leafy green vegetables and cereal grains for K. Here, too, Vitamin K is stored for future use, so you don't need it every day. There is some evidence that Vitamin K can interfere with the anti-clotting effects of blood thinners, so if that's a specific issue in your case, talk with your caregiver.

Calcium

We all know how wonderful calcium is when it comes to building and maintaining strong bones and teeth. But did you know it also helps regulate muscle contractions (like your heart), and helps blood clot? A lack of calcium is a serious thing; it's called rickets in children and osteoporosis in adults. Something else we all know: You can find plenty of calcium in milk, cheese, and other dairy foods...but did you know it's also in leafy green vegetables, soy beans, nuts, and even fish like sardines—the fish where you eat the bone, of course. Too much calcium, however, isn't so great; it can lead to stomach pain and diarrhea and might contribute to kidney stones.

Iodine

Iodine helps your thyroid function and helps your cells work properly, too. Sea fish, shellfish, even some plant foods have iodine, depending on where and in what soil that plant is grown. But you'll also find that iodine has been added to standard table salt for more than half a century with no ill effects and plenty of benefits. But be careful, megadosing beyond normal consumption levels could negatively affect your thyroid gland and lead to weight gain. Nobody wants that.

Potassium

Potassium helps control the balance of fluids in your body and helps the heart. You'll find it in bananas and other fruits, some vegetables, nuts, and fish, beef, and poultry. And you may need less of it as you get older, as your kidney becomes less able to process and remove potassium from your system. Too much potassium can cause stomach pain and diarrhea. In fact, older people shouldn't take potassium supplements unless they're advised to do so by their doctors.

Iron

Just like calcium, iron is one of the best known of the body's minerals. It makes red blood cells and a deficiency is well known as *anemia*. You'll find it in meats, yes, but also in beans, nuts, and dried fruits, and in dark-green leafy vegetables like watercress and kale; so even if you're a low- or no-meat-eater, it's readily available. There are some drawbacks to overdosing, however: Taking over twenty milligrams of iron—which is a lot!—can cause constipation, stomach pain, and vomiting. Very high doses can actually be fatal, especially in children. Another reason not to have supplements lying around the house.

Salt

Salt is a pesky one. We do need it—about six grams of salt a day (that's twenty-four grams of sodium—and "salt" and "sodium" are different substances, and shouldn't be confused). That's around a teaspoon. Children, obviously, need less, and babies none at all (their kidneys aren't ready for it).

America's biggest problem with salt is that we use way too much of it. Not just table salt—in fact, table salt is a minor offender in the real world. Its presence in the food itself—in snack foods, in processed foods, in pickled and preserved foods, in almost *everything* that's a common part of the American diet—is so huge that we all take in many times the recommended dose of salt every day. And removing it from your diet is not only *not* recommended (you do need it)…it's damn near impossible. Salt *reduction* is possible, and a worthwhile pursuit, but removal? It can't and shouldn't happen.

Cutting salty snacks and most or all highly processed foods out of your regular diet will help a great deal. Checking on salt or sodium contents in your favorite foods is also a good idea—and don't rely just on the package labels, they are often intentionally and unintentionally misleading. Any of the good eating apps for your phones are better. It is, in fact, the closest thing we have to a "miracle" drug. It makes food taste better, even in the tiniest quantities; it helps your body retain water and function more efficiently. But by the same token, too much salt can cause an increase in blood pressure in many people (not all; maybe only as much as half the population, but we have no way of knowing *which* half is salt-sensitive at the moment), cause you to retain water, and wreak havoc on your system overall.

A switch in eating patterns to personally prepared rather than processed foods and the replacement of salty snacks with fruits and vegetables will do wonders. And please, don't bother with the heavily marketed "salt substitutes." That's just exchanging one set of chemicals for others that we know even less about, and they generally taste like metal shavings. Garlic, on the other hand, is a great substitute, as are many chilis and onion derivatives. Go for spice, not salt, and you'll be surprised how quickly you find over-salted foods unappealing. They'll start to burn your tongue and bother your belly...and that's where you want to be.

You get the idea. There is a long list of other "trace elements"—chromium, cobalt, copper, and on and on—that you need as well. Even ominous-sounding ones like phosphorus and molybdenum. But you can easily see the pattern that emerges just from the ones we have so briefly discussed: *A diet rich in fruits and vegetables, especially leafy greens, that emphasizes fish over red meat and relies on fiber will give you all the vitamins you need without worries about overdose.* In other words, supplements aren't necessary, are occasionally hazardous, and are a $30 billion dollar drain on your bank account.

And of course there are some exceptions.

For all of their overuse, vitamin and mineral supplements aren't all bad—few things in The Land of Healthcare are (with the exception of tobacco). Supplements can play an important role for some particular groups who are at high risk.

- People with osteoporosis, especially older people, may require extra vitamin D and calcium.
- People with Crohn's disease or celiac disease have difficulty absorbing some vitamins and minerals.
- People with vitamin B12 deficiency almost always need a supplement.
- People who have undergone particular kinds of bariatric surgery for weight loss, like the gastric sleeve, actually lose the ability to absorb vitamins and minerals at

"normal" rates and should be taking vitamin supplements for the rest of their lives to remain healthy (that's a consequence of weight-loss surgery you don't hear too much about until after the surgery's taken place, unfortunately).

But these are exceptions to the rule. For the vast majority of us even minimally healthy Americans, even those eating a far less-than-perfect diet…supplements just aren't necessary.

The Elephant in the Room: Vitamin D

Like every great rule, there is one possible, *possible* reason for modern Americans to consider the use of a specific vitamin supplement: Vitamin D.

Vitamin D isn't technically a vitamin at all, it's a "prohormone," a string of molecules on its way to becoming a hormone. It is vital and very beneficial for the human body. Among other things, Vitamin D helps with the immune system, the brain, and the nervous system, supports lung function, regulates the amount of calcium and phosphate in the body—which leads to healthy bones and teeth—and is a major tool in regulating insulin and therefore helping with diabetes management. It might even help prevent cancer or diabetes, but there need to be larger, more reliable studies to confirm that.

There is some disagreement about minimum doses per day or week, but generally speaking, experts agree that fifteen micrograms a day is good for adults, and a little bit more if you're past seventy. Overdose of Vitamin D is unlikely, but if you get too ambitious too much over a long period of time and consume 4,000 or more micrograms on a regular basis, it could result in a build-up of calcium, which can actually *weaken* bones rather than *strengthen* them, as well as damage the heart and kidney. So where fifteen

---

micrograms a day might be a good idea, one hundred micrograms a day could be harmful.

But really…we don't get enough of it. In the testing of large populations, researchers found a startling deficiency in Vitamin D; so much so that the government actually suggests a daily supplement containing ten micrograms to be taken during autumn and winter. Your age, weight, and liver and kidney function can affect your D requirements as well.

Vitamin D deficiency isn't a minor thing either. Experts ascribe a lack of D to everything from frequent illness and fatigue to back pain, muscle pain, and reduced ability to heal wounds. A long-term deficiency may be even worse, with possible complications for your heart, your brain, and your autoimmune system. It can cause bone conditions such as rickets and osteoporosis.

Most of the Vitamin D your body needs is derived from direct sunlight on the skin when you're outdoors (the UV-B rays that trigger Vitamin D production can't pass through clothing, glass, or plastic, so outdoors it is). It *is* possible to get at least some of your D from foods. The University of Florida (check the resources section at the end of the book) points out that some common foods can help load you up appropriately. For example:

- 3 ounces of cooked sockeye salmon:(14 mcg)
- 3 ounces of drained canned tuna (6 mcg)
- 3 ounces of drained canned sardines (4 mcg)
- 1 cup of 1% fortified milk (3 mcg)
- A hard-boiled egg (1 mcg)

And Vitamin D has been added to many common foods, especially spreads and cereals and cow milk. Though really, the sun is the thing.

And therein lies the problem. Most of us modern Western twenty-first century people don't get nearly enough sunlight to make the Vitamin D we need. And even if you're getting a moderate amount of sun, other factors can control your level of absorption, from geography to skin color to time of year.

And then, of course, there's sunscreen.

Anyone who's concerned about the potential for skin cancer has heard the mantra many times: even small exposure to the sun can increase your risk for melanoma. On the other hand, doctors and nutritionists tell us we *need* exposure to that very same sun to get the minimum amount of vitamin D our body requires.

Once again, we're back to that "mindfulness" thing. Generally speaking, the balance seems to be *ten to fifteen minutes of sun, at least two or three times a week* for a person with light skin, and up *to two hours a day* for a person with dark skin. As a general rule of thumb, many healthcare providers advise that you say in the sun for about half as long as it takes you to burn, and that generally speaking the early morning hours are the best time to get all the UV-B you need without worrying about a burn. Easier said than done for many of us, but there you go.

Given all these complexities and the complications of modern life, you can see why a daily supplement of fifteen micrograms makes sense for most of us.

Maybe. If you're concerned about this one, once again, talk to your caregiver. Getting a test for D deficiency isn't expensive or painful, and might be covered by your insurance. And if you find out your diet and exposure is fine, that's another place you can save money—far more than the cost of a blood test every now and then to make sure you're doing things right. Meanwhile: more sun! More salmon! More tuna! More hard-boiled eggs!

MONITORING YOUR SLEEP

**Jack Dorsey has a wearable sleep monitor
that measures sleep quality, recovery speed, and daily
activity. "If I keep to a consistent schedule of sleep, I get
higher scores on REM and I get much deeper sleep as well."**

N o matter how far afield we may roam, we always come
back to this one central principle: *mindfulness.* Jack
Dorsey preaches it and practices it with every one of
his suggestions, and sleep is no exception.

Of all the healthful practices we've talked about here—
activity, eating patterns, peace of mind, and the rest—nothing
is more underestimated or just plain overlooked than *sleep.* So
let's take a few minutes to talk about it: what it is, how important it is, and how you can get better at it. Then we'll talk about
a couple of different ways you can monitor it and improve your
quality of sleep—as you should.

Why Sleep Matters So Much

Your muscles and metabolism aren't the only parts of you that need rest. Your entire being needs *and deserves* some time off, and sleep is as essential for your mind and soul as it is for your meat and bones. This isn't just good spiritual advice; this comes from scientists as well. Let's quickly run down the Golden List of Benefits from Sleep:

- **Cognition, productivity, and concentration**
- **Calorie regulation.** The need to consume fewer calories during the day.
- **Better athletic performance.** Including better performance on the walking and HIIT goals that Jack Dorsey sets for himself and you may want to set for yourself as well. (Generally speaking, highly successful athletes sleep a couple of hours more a night compared to us normal humans)
- **Lower risk of heart disease.** A wide range of studies have confirmed this over and over.
- **Improved autoimmune response.** Simply put: You don't get sick as often or as seriously when your immune system is working its best, and sleep is essential to that optimum performance
- **Lower inflammation.** It may be the buzzword of the twenty-first century, but it's true: Inflammation can badly affect your ability to heal, to grow, and to stay healthy…and consistently good sleep lowers your level of inflammation body-wide.

- **Depression prevention (and all that implies).** No less a trusted source than the *Journal of the American Medical Association* has told us that lack of sleep is a contributing factor to death by suicide.

Basically, sleep affects every part of your body and mind. Dr. Michael Twery, a sleep expert at the National Institutes of Health, said in a recent NIH article that sleep affects "growth and stress hormones, our immune system, appetite, breathing, blood pressure, and cardiovascular health."

Do you need other reasons? That isn't enough? Okay, look at it the other way around. Here's what you're risking if you *don't* get adequate high-quality sleep:

- Obesity
- Heart disease
- Infection
- Blood pressure
- Blood sugar control

It can even induce diabetes-like symptoms and may even affect how well vaccinations work in your body. So...get serious about it.

High-quality Sleep is the Only Worthwhile Sleep

A good night's sleep consists of four to five sleep cycles, and each cycle includes periods of light sleep, deep sleep, and our old friend REM—not the rock and roll band, but the original REM: "Rapid Eye Movement," the time when you dream. "As the night goes on, the portion of that cycle that is in REM sleep increases. It turns out that this pattern of cycling and progression is critical to the biology of sleep," Dr. Twery of the NIH tells us.

How much sleep do you need? It varies as you get older, but on average, almost all experts agree you need at least seven to eight hours of sleep a night. And the *quality* of sleep is important as well—vitally so. As often as humanly possible, sleep should be uninterrupted and undisturbed by extraneous light, noises, stimulants, and physical discomfort (in English: an uncomfortable bed).

Two of the most common and most insidious enemies of high-quality sleep are *insomnia* and *apnea*.

Insomnia, as we all know, is simply the inability to sleep and sleep well. We all suffer from it now and then—it is the modern world, after all—but a consistent state of low-quality sleep or sleeplessness is physically dangerous.

Apnea is a physical condition in which your breathing is irregular or interrupted while you sleep. It can be due to a lot of things, including your weight and the physical structure of your throat and mouth.

We won't go into great detail here—these are serious conditions, but their causes and treatment differ radically from person to person. The take-home message, however, is clear: If you're suffering from insomnia, or if you snore loudly and often—so loudly it disturbs other people in your home, so often it wakes you multiple times every night—*get to a qualified healthcare provider and do something about it.* Your health—your *life*—is at stake.

But if it's not that serious—if you're like most of us and you simply have trouble getting to sleep or staying asleep more than you like, and/or if you don't feel rested when you get up the next day...there are things you can do to change that.

How to Sleep Better

Here are just a few common-sense strategies:

- Go to bed around the same time each night. It sounds silly, but it's true; your body responds well to *patterns of behavior*, and this is an important one. For all the distractions from family community and the internet, try to go to bed and keep a consistent "sleepy time" schedule.
- Spend more time outside during the day.
- Avoid sleeping in when you have already had enough sleep.
- Get a comfortable bed. Seriously. If your mattress is lumpy, if it's developed a "well" in the middle, or if it just doesn't suit you anymore (or never did)...invest the time and money and change it. Make your bed a place you *want* to spend eight or nine hours out of every twenty-four.
- Avoid a large meal within a couple of hours of bedtime.
- Stop imbibing alcohol a couple of hours before bed time. It may help you *get* to sleep, but it seriously damages the *quality* of the sleep you'll have.

- A warm bath can actually help.
- Reduce uncertainty and anxiety about the next day by spending a few minutes writing up a "to do" list, so you know what's ahead.
- Many people swear by yoga or meditation (see our earlier chapter on those healthful approaches to life and thought).
- Read or listen to music or environmentally-based "white noise."
- DON'T interact with your phone, the news, or social media.
- Reduce extraneous light and noise as much as you can. Consider blackout curtains, low-cost sound insulation, or even moving your sleep area to a quieter part of your home.
- Cut out caffeine at least four hours before bed time (or cut it out entirely if you know it's a sleep disruptor for you). And not just coffee: most soft drinks, cocoa, and even chocolate have caffeine as well.
- Stop smoking. Of course. But in this case in particular, because nicotine is a stimulant that is a proven enemy of sleep.
- If you can't sleep…get up. Do something. But do something *relaxing*, whether it's reading or knitting or meditating. Don't go back to work and don't go online. That will only make matters worse.
- Keep a sleep journal.

A Sleep Journal Can Help

Simply being aware of how important sleep is, and how well you're sleeping, can help you get better rest. Jack Dorsey prefers a device—an Oura Ring, at last report—and we'll talk about other sleep monitoring apps, pro and con. But the goal of *mindfulness* can be reached in a number of ways.

You might want to start with a simple pen-and-paper Sleep Journal. You can make up a nice little chart you can keep on the wall or near your bed, or you can jot down the answer to these questions every morning in your life journal or a ready-made notebook. It doesn't matter…but it should be *written*, not an artifact of memory, and it should be filled out *daily*, not once in a while when you think you remember what happened. Once again: Make it a regular routine to help with *mindfulness*.

Here are the questions you should be asking yourself, and the answers you should be recording:

1. What time did you go to bed last night?
2. How long did it take you to fall asleep (approximately; don't watch the clock!)?
3. How many times did you wake up during the night?
4. If you did wake up, how long were you awake, total, during the night?
5. When did you finally wake up?
6. What were your total number of hours asleep (rounded to the quarter hour)?
7. When did you *get* up (and there is no wrong answer; some of us like to "lounge.")?

8. How would you rate the quality of your sleep last night?
9. How did you feel in the morning? Refreshed? Fatigued? Try to rate it on a one-to-ten scale.
10. Did you feel it necessary, or even preferable, to take a nap during the day?

The first thing the sleep journal will do is give you a practical, objective record of how well you're sleeping, and if there's room for improvement. When you've got that picture clear, you can employ as many of the "better sleep" tips listed above as you like—including, if necessary, a trip to a sleep specialist—and then *keep on keeping the diary*. Now you have a baseline, and a way to quantitatively measure your improvement...as well as something to celebrate as your sleep habits improve. And all this is possible without a smart phone in sight.

There's an App for That

Of course there is. There are a huge number of activity trackers and sleep trackers available, for free and for a few bucks, as well as actual devices like the Oura Ring, that can give you even more information.

Some humans thrive on numbers. It gives them something to compare to, a way to set goals and to appreciate improvement. They are motivating, but those same set of numbers (and the tools that provide them) can be over-complicating and even counter-productive for others, who see all that data as a burden and a constant reminder that they're not doing enough.

Maybe it's time to figure out which kind of person you are. There are plenty of non-invasive, even gentle, but still useful tools that can help you measure and improve your sleep. *Monitoring* is the important part. *How* you monitor is entirely up to you and your own personal preferences. Isn't it liberating to know there are no wrong answers?

Many of the wearable trackers are like old-fashioned wrist watches; other can be clipped to your pillow or can sit on the table beside your bed.

Among many other thing, most sleep trackers measure:

- **Duration of sleep,** including when you fall asleep and when you wake up.
- **Quality of sleep,** including interruptions, waking, and even tossing and turning.
- **Sleep phases,** like REM and deep sleep—other important factors in assessing the quality of your slumber.
- **Your sleep environment,** like how dark and quiet your room is, what the temperature is, and how those change during your sleepy-time.
- **Other factors that can affect your sleep,** like recent consumption of calories, alcohol, caffeine, or even your stress levels.

Keep in mind, though, that sleep trackers don't actually measure your sleep *directly.* They're really just guesstimating how much you actually sleeping based on your body's lack of movement. This information can be a great help, just like a sleep journal, when you are assessing your current, "baseline" sleep quality; these insights can point you towards what to do to improve it, but don't mistake it for solid scientific data. This isn't a *program;* it's just *information,* and it's still up to you to interpret it and act on it. Real scientific data and reliable advice is only available through a sleep study at an accredited institution, where your brain waves and breathing are monitoring constantly during a full night's sleep. (And if your primary care provider or specialist sees signs of apnea or other sleep disorders, they will recommend you to one of the growing number of sleep centers available now. The amount of information you receive from this research is awesome.)

Makers of sleep tech and scientists can agree on one thing: Sleep-tracking apps and devices can be useful for getting a broad look at your sleep, but people should resist drawing conclusions about their sleep health.

Sleep Well

Your brain and body exist on the planet a full twenty-four hours a day, and—if you're doing something right—nearly a third of that time is spent *sleeping.* So pay attention to that state of being as closely as you pay attention to your more conscious hours. Think about it. Assess it objectively. And, if necessary, work to improve it. It will make the other sixteen (or so) hours a day so much better…and you'll be around longer to enjoy them.

JOURNALING

Dorsey writes about his day on the Notes app on his iPhone. "I try to do that every single day, usually when I'm wrapping up the day,"

We're going to finish this exploration into the Jack Dorsey Way of living a healthy, productive, energetic life with the most personal practice of all: keeping a journal.

It's an activity that has been with us for as long as literacy itself. Many of our greatest historical documents are journals or diaries. Some of the greatest novels of western civilization, from *Dracula* to *The Color Purple,* were written as diaries, daybooks, or letters.

As a personal pursuit, journaling fell out of favor for everyone but thirteen-year-old-girls for a few decades of the twentieth century, but it's made a recent comeback for people of all ages who are seeking balance, personal insight, and a regular opportunity for introspection. Maybe the whole concept of blogging, from the early days of LiveJournal and MySpace to the full-frontal assault of Facebook, has repopularized the idea, or maybe it's always been something special for humans that was just temporarily underappreciated. Cultural rhythms aside, today we find that journaling is something that everyone from teachers to authors to spiritual leaders to CEOs praise and rely on.

And yes, there is a growing body of scientific research that affirms the power and importance of the practice. Commonly referred to as "therapeutic journaling," it has become a common recommendation for counselors and psychiatrists of every stripe.

Psychologist Shilagh Mirgain, in a recent interview, said therapeutic journaling uses the written word, "to express the full range of emotions we may have related to difficult or traumatic life events. In doing so, we can help create a greater sense of well-being." Researchers at institutions from Harvard to the University of Rochester have supported the hypothesis that journaling provides a number of unique and powerful benefits. The list is long and impressive:

Journaling helps with anxiety and stress, as well as depression. Michigan State University cites a study published in *Psychological Science* that noted how writing down your thoughts and then physically throwing away the paper you wrote them on can be an effective way to clear your mind. A wide range of other studies show that giving "voice" to your biggest concerns or fears, envisioning your greatest hopes and ambitions, and simply relieving the pressure of what is currently, overwhelmingly *bothering* you can lead—if properly channeled—to insight and new energy. Reductions in anxiety lead directly to physical benefits, like more and better sleep, better eating and activity habits, and an improvement in cognitive abilities. Quite simply, a happy and tranquil mind *thinks better,* and journaling is a proven, valuable tool to reach that objective.

Journaling can help you set and achieve goals, both personal and professional. Writing something down tells you brain that *this is important.* Neuroscientists refer to it as your *reticular activating system,* and "cementing" it in your cortex actually increases the likelihood of remembering and achieving those goals. This is distinctly different (or should be) than the keeping and updating of a daily or weekly "To Do" list. That is a separate tool that can work beautifully for some people, and be nothing but a burden and emotional weight for others. In journaling, the goal is much wider. It's most productive in this context when it is used to confront the larger issues of what you would like to be doing, where you would like to *be,* both physically and mentally, in the future. Detail is good. Dreaming is required. *Knowing yourself* is the goal.

Journaling can help improve your memory. Obviously the beneficial process of RAS works on the much more practical, not to mention essential, function of simply *remembering things.* Writing down names, experiences, the results of important interactions—with other people, other entities, and the world at large—creates a more "solid" and retrievable memory. It's why we take notes in school and meetings, and we why keep "to do" lists. This can apply to your emotional well-being as much as your organizational skills.

Journaling can improve your communication skills. A surprising, though not entirely illogical, benefit of journaling could be an improvement in your storytelling and communications skills—very valuable tools in your "other" professional and personal pursuits. Decades ago, Stanford researcher Melanie Sperling offered the truism that "writing and speaking are critically linked" and pointed out how the subvocalization of tracing your written thoughts naturally translates into actual vocalization. As you tell stories to yourself, as you try to express your most important thoughts to yourself, you're actually building up a set of "best practices" on how to do exactly the same with others, so the next time you want or need to tell a story, or to express yourself fully, passionately, and compellingly, all those hours of journaling will inform your process.

Journaling can improve your creativity. Julia Cameron's *The Artist's Way* has been enhancing and triggering the creative process for decades—about four million times over. Journaling has always been an important part of the Artist's Way, especially Cameron's "Morning Pages" tactic—the process of writing without thinking, producing at least three pages of "stream of consciousness" writing every morning. Check our Resources section for more information on her invaluable book and her website as well, if creative "juice" is one of your goals. She is far from alone; teachers of writing, art, and spiritual fulfillment agree that ideas flow more easily from a mind at rest, and often occur at times when you are not "working" directly on the problem: in the shower, on a walk…or when journaling.

Journaling can help improve or enhance your emotional intelligence. "Emotional Intelligence" is the ability to perceive and manage emotions—your own and those of others. Journaling can help you process those emotions and increase your self-awareness of the internal lives of other people as well as your own. And once you begin to understand *other* people's reasons for their behavior, you can take a big step towards interacting with them in a much healthier way.

Journaling can help you heal… and not just emotionally. A wide range of studies have shown that journaling can improve your physical health as well. Clearly, journaling provides a valuable tool for tracking day-to-day symptoms of chronic conditions and chronic pain, and it serves as an aid for better management. Additionally, a study published in 2006 in the *Journal of the American Medical Association* found that patients struggling with a chronic illness who wrote down their thoughts about stressful situations actually experienced fewer physical symptoms than patients who did not journal. And research shows similar results in the treatment of eating disorders, bipolar disorders, and even schizophrenia. Meanwhile, the *Telegraph* reported that researchers at the University of Arizona found keeping a journal after a divorce resulted in lower heart rates and higher "heart rate variability"—a factor that is associated with better health. No less a light than Dr. James

Pennebaker, author of *Opening Up by Writing It Down* (check our Resources sections for more information), reports that journaling strengthens immune cells—the ones called T-lymphocytes. How much all of this is connected or enhanced by the proven effects of journaling on stress reduction is unclear, but ultimately...does it matter? It's pretty obvious, and has been frequently confirmed, that journaling is good for you, body and soul.

Psychologists, counselors, and many mental health professionals use journaling techniques every day to accomplish all of the above and much more. Even primary care providers and healthcare specialists use journaling to help their patients deal with chronic conditions like arthritis, cancer, diabetes, asthma and other progressive or recurring conditions. It's proven—*proven*—to be an effective way to track symptoms and to provide a valuable tactic in discovering new ways to cope with the challenges these people face.

And you don't need to be deeply unhappy or disturbed to benefit from journaling. Quite the contrary; its values are available even to highly motivated and successful people—like Jack Dorsey—who have found repeatedly that there is more to learn and enjoy even in a very full life, when you build moments of self-reflection and "pause" into your busy life.

How to Journal

There isn't a strict rulebook for journaling—in fact, there shouldn't be. It is among the most personal tasks you'll ever undertake. There are some "best practices" that seem to work well for the vast majority of people who journal, and some frequently asked questions that people new to journaling need answers to.

How much and how often? You'd be surprised at how little is effective (similar to the benefits that can be derived from even a little exercise, meditative time, or additional sleep). "Just 20 minutes at a time over four consecutive days was associated with a decrease in health problems, such as enhancing the immune system functioning," Shilagh Mirgain noted in a 2016 interview. Other research has found that writing about meaningful personal experiences for as little as fifteen minutes a day on a regular basis can help with everything from a sense of personal satisfaction to better grades in school. Even as little as *four minutes a day* can have a measurable impact.

Be consistent. This comes up over and over again. Virtually all the experts agree: Try to write every day, especially when you first begin journaling. You'll find—like all good habits—it becomes a bit addictive after a while; you'll feel "off" when you don't. But at first, make it a daily practice, preferably at the same time every day, when you can structure ten minutes to half an hour as quiet and uninterrupted (or uninterruptable). That's easier said than done in a busy life, it's true, but it's worth it.

What should I write about? The tempting answer is, "anything you want," and to the degree that you should let words and thoughts flow freely…that's true. On the other hand, many guides to beneficial journaling urge you to go beyond simply recounting daily events, and sticking to subjects that are truly important to you. If there has been a conflict at work or at the home that needs examination, here's the place. But remember to apply the same attention to triumphs or advances in your life as well. And remember to *move on*, regardless. Your life, both internal and external, is about far more than just one thing, one relationship, one situation. If you find yourself writing about the same subject three or four days in a row, consider putting that topic aside for a few weeks and looking in other directions instead. And don't feel as if every entry has to be transformative or revelatory. You may think you *have* to write about some deep, dark thing that is bothering you every single day…but you don't. Not always. And if that examination or revisitation is truly upsetting, let it rest until it really *is* the right time to talk about it, even to yourself.

At base: *Learn to trust yourself,* and that inner voice you've always had, the one you're trying to bring forward, maybe for the first time. Just keep in mind: There's no hurry. You'll be doing this every day. It's all good.

Plan on keeping it private. You can keep these pages (physical or digital) for years and re-read them at will, or you can rip them up and throw them away the day they're done. Move forward with the thought that it is entirely private and personal: This is only for you, not for anyone else. So you don't have to worry about spelling and grammar, you don't have to worry about offending or frightening anyone.

If you happen on some revelation or gem you do want to share, you can—but keep it to a fragment, expressed away from the journal itself. This is *yours*, as personal and private as your own thoughts.

One Word of Caution

It's the same word of caution we've expressed in almost every other chapter: *moderation.* Journaling is a valuable tool, but it is only that: a *tool*, not a way of life. So here are a few quick tips:

Know when to stop. Keep it to your allotted period of time—fifteen minutes, twenty minute, half an hour. Then *stop.* If you're in the middle of an important thought, you can break off, knowing you will remember what you were saying when you pick it up the next day. And if you can't... consider the possibility that it wasn't all that important a thought after all.

Don't stop early. At the other end of the spectrum, there will be days when you don't have anything particularly interesting to stay...but journal anyway. Feel free to repeat yourself. Talk about how you don't have anything to say. It really doesn't matter; it will all work out in the end. But keep at it for the allotted time.

Sometimes it may make you sad, and that's okay. Many people who are new to journaling report that they often feel blue or depressed, but in most cases that passes quickly, as they experience insight, joy, and melancholy in equal measure.

And if upset or depression after journaling persists, STOP. Every proponent of the method will tell you the same thing: journaling is not for everyone. Psychologists and psychiatrists who employ it know this, and they keep a lookout for signs that it's doing more harm than good—manifestations like hypervigilance, obsessive thoughts, mounting stress or distress. If you feel you're experiencing any of these, then journaling may be a trigger that's taking you in an unhealthy direction, and it's time to talk to a qualified psychologist, counselor or healthcare provider.

Tools for Journaling

One last thing: *There's no wrong way to do it.* Sometimes you'll hear or read about how much *better* journaling in longhand is, or how a particularly bound book or page format is the *best*. This is just nonsense. *How* you journal is as personal a decision, based on personal preference, as what your journal is *about*.

If you're someone who rarely writes with a paper and pen and finds, instead, that your smartphone is your most preferred and enjoyable form of communication, then use one of the many phone apps that are available. That's what Jack Dorsey does. He uses Notes on his iPhone for his daily journal. "It's searchable. It's accessible all the time. It's in the cloud, so I can get to it even if I don't have my phone. It's secure."

If you come from a tradition or generation that is most comfortable with a keyboard, journal on your laptop or tablet, where your thoughts can flow fast and free.

And if you're the type, of any age, who loves the feel of a pen or pencil in your hand and paper under our fingertips, then by all mean, *write*. There are a nearly infinite number of beautiful writing instruments and journals available at any stationery store, online or brick-and mortar.

It doesn't matter. What matters is that you *do* it—at least *try* it. Give it a couple of weeks of daily attention, at the minimum. Get past the temporary discomfort of a "permanent" change in schedule, and see where journaling leads you.

You maybe be pleasantly surprised at what you find. And that's all part of the Jack Dorsey Way.

Words to Live By

Let's end this section—and this book—with something very appropriate: *words*. In this case, words about journaling itself.

We began this chapter talking about how great writers, great thinkers, and great historians have been using journals and diaries for centuries. It's not surprising, then, that many of them occasionally wrote about journaling itself. Maybe these quick quotes will inspire you to give it a try...

"In the journal I do not just express myself more openly than I could to any person; I create myself."

—*Susan Sontag*

"The only thing I have done religiously in my life is keep a journal, I have hundreds of them, filled with feathers, flowers, photographs, and words—without locks, open on my shelves."

—*Terry Tempest Williams*

"Journaling is like whispering to one's self and listening at the same time."

—*Mina Murray*

"People who keep journals have life twice."

—*Jessamyn West*

"Keeping a journal of what's going on in your life is a good way to help you distill what's important and what's not."

—*Martina Navratilova*

"In the journal I am at ease."

—*Anais Nin*

"I can shake off everything as I write; my sorrows disappear, my courage is reborn."

—*Anne Frank*

"I've always written. There's a journal which I kept from about 9 years old."

—*Maya Angelou*

"Your subconscious mind is trying to help you all the time. That's why I keep a journal—not for chatter but for mostly the images that flow into the mind or little ideas. I keep a running journal, and I have all of my life, so it's like your gold mine when you start writing."

—*Jim Harrison*

"I don't journal to 'be productive.' I don't do it to find great ideas or to put down prose I can later publish. The pages aren't intended for anyone but me. It's the most cost-effective therapy I've ever found."

—*Tim Ferriss*

"Fill your paper with the breathings of your heart."

—*William Wordsworth*

"As there are a thousand thoughts lying within a man that he does not know till he takes up the pen to write."

—*William Makepeace Thackeray*

"I never travel without my diary. One should always have something sensational to read on the train."

—*Oscar Wilde*

A FINAL WORD

When you first look at Jack Dorsey's multifaceted way of life, it seems a little...*scattered*. Walking, workouts, fasting, meditation—it seems to be a little bit of everything, thrown into one very demanding and slightly odd-shaped sack.

But the more you dig into it, the more you find an unexpected and almost uplifting unity. Jack Dorsey is looking at the *whole* of his life, from physical activity to mental acuity to spiritual centeredness, as a single unified *thing*, an artifact that he believes is remarkably malleable, *improvable*, and very largely under his control.

It's hard to disagree with a man who began in relative obscurity and built a life-changing tool and a whole new culture in just a few short years. He *is* a man who has learned how to harness a great deal of his potential, and for all his eccentricities and extremes—and let's be clear, there is nothing *not* extreme about OMAD and weekend fast—it's clear he has something important to tell us. It's not terribly surprising that many of these lessons are ones we've heard from fitness experts, spiritual advisers, self-help "gurus," and our wise ol' family practitioners for our entire lives:

Eat better.
Get more exercise.
Treat your body and your mind with the
care and respect they deserve.
Work on your inner self as hard as your outer self.
All things in moderation.
Mindfulness.

Hopefully going through these strategies, learning more about each of them and how they might affect or improve your life, has been both informative and a little inspiring. Now is the time to go back to that first chapter—the one on *How to Use This Book*—and think once again about what's important to you. What are your own goals? What would you like to improve? And how much time, energy, and focus can you *truly* dedicate to changing yourself for the better—starting right now.

You don't have to do everything at once. That's obvious. Jack Dorsey himself didn't create his very demanding daily and weekly routine in a sudden overnight flash. It is the product of years of experimentation, adventure, and trial-and-error, and it continues to change on a regular—or rather, an *irregular*—basis. Yours will probably do the same. But there should be something, somewhere, in these pages that interest you, intrigues you, or sets your mind spinning.

Grab that. Do that thing. Get started. Not just (or at all) because Jack Dorsey does it or says you should. Do it because it's something *you* want to do, for yourself and for the people you care about.

Time to change the world—*your* world.

Time to get started.

RESOURCES

About Jack Dorsey:

A good summary of these habits from the CNBC website: https://www.cnbc.com/2019/04/08/twitter-and-square-ceo-jack-dorsey-on-his-personal-wellness-habits.html

The Atlantic's approach is slightly more combative and cynical, but grudgingly admits it's probably not entirely crazy: https://www.theatlantic.com/health/archive/2019/01/silicon-valley-extreme-diets-fasting/681566/

On Meditation:

Nine Meditation Teachers You Should Know: https://www.yogajournal.com/meditation/9-meditation-teachers-know

The books of Pema Chodron are a great plain-language introduction to the basics of meditation. Start with *When Things Fall Apart* or *Comfortable with Uncertainty*

"The Daily Habits of Successful People": https://www.huffpost.com/entry/business-meditation-executives-meditate_n_3528731

Different types of meditation may have different effects: https://www.ncbi.nlm.nih.gov/pmc/articles/PMC1697747/

The scientific basis of meditation: https://nccih.nih.gov/health/meditation/overview.htm

Healthline's revealing article on the different types of meditation: https://www.healthline.com/health/mental-health/types-of-meditation

The benefits of meditation: https://www.healthline.com/nutrition/12-benefits-of-meditation#section1

A great piece from *The Huffington Post* on pain control and meditation: https://www.huffpost.com/entry/meditation-health-benefits_n_3178731?utm_hp_ref=mostpopular

Positive Psychology's extensive piece on the history of meditation: https://positivepsychology.com/history-of-meditation/

Details on *Vipassanā* meditation: https://www.dhamma.org/en-US/index

An alphabetical list alphabetical list of worldwide *Vipassanā* course: https://www.dhamma.org/en-US/locations/directory

More from Meditation Advisor Lodro Rinzler: https://www.sonima.com/author/lodro-rinzler/

On Walking:

Walking can spark creativity. A 2014 study from the *Journal of Experimental Psychology*. https://www.apa.org/pubs/journals/releases/xlm-a0036577.pdf

A study published in the British *Journal of Sports Medicine* found that those who adhered to a walking program showed significant improvements in blood pressure, slowing of resting heart rate, reduction of body fat and body weight, reduced cholesterol, improved depression scores with better quality of life, and increased measures of endurance. https://bjsm.bmj.com/content/49/11/710

More on *Walk Your Way to Better Health*, by Michele Staten, a walking coach, from the usually pretty reliable *Prevention* Magazine: https://order.hearstproducts.com/subscribe/hstproducts/250921?source=_cd_&utm_campaign=_ed_&utm_content=a20485587&utm_medium=referral&utm_source=prevention.com

Walking benefits everyone, regardless of age, gender, or fitness level. Here's an abstract from a talk given at EuroPrevent 2019, an event from the European Society of Cardiology: https://esc365.escardio.org/Congress/EuroPrevent-2019/Rapid-Fire-Session-2/190462-sex-and-age-specific-associations-between-cardiorespiratory-fitness-cvd-morbidity-and-all-cause-mortality-in-316-137-swedish-adults#abstract

How walking can help with joint pain. An April 2019 study from the *American Journal of Preventive Medicine*: https://www.ajpmonline.org/article/S0749-3797(19)30045-5/fulltext

An abstract on a study that shows how just twelve minutes of walking can increase joviality, vigor, attentiveness and self-confidence: https://www.ncbi.nlm.nih.gov/pubmed/27100368

A fascinating study from the *Journal of Experimental Psychology, Learning, Memory, and Cognition* on how going for a walk can spark creativity: https://www.apa.org/pubs/journals/releases/xlm-a0036577.pdf

One possible 30-minute "walking workout" to use on your treadmill, from NBC News: https://www.nbcnews.com/better/health/30-minute-treadmill-workout-no-running-required-ncna797811

On High-Intensity Interval Training (HIIT):

The original HIIT Plan from the American College of Sports Medicine: https://journals.lww.com/acsm-healthfitness/Fulltext/2013/05000/HIGH_INTENSITY_CIRCUIT_TRAINING_USING_BODY_WEIGHT_.5.aspx

A set of HIIT workouts from *Men's Journal*: https://www.mensjournal.com/tag/high-intensity-workouts

A study that shows how people prefer HIIT to other high-intensity workouts: https://www.ncbi.nlm.nih.gov/pubmed/25486273

On Ice Baths and Saunas:

The Atlantic explains how saunas can't "detoxify" your body: https://www.theatlantic.com/health/archive/2017/06/infrared-saunas-will-not-detoxify-you-toxins-sweat/528813/

The basics of hyperthermia from the Society of Thermal Medicine: https://www.thermaltherapy.org/ebusSFTM/SOCIETYINFO/WhatisThermalMedicine.aspx

A piece on how cold showers can be used as a treatment for depression from the NCBI: https://www.ncbi.nlm.nih.gov/pubmed/17993252

A podcast with Dr. Rhonda Patrick on the benefits of saunas: https://biohackersummit.com/2016/11/10/dr-rhonda-patrick-nutritional-health-benefits-sauna/

An article from *The Guardian* on how saunas help us live longer: https://www.theguardian.com/lifeandstyle/2015/feb/23/saunas-help-you-live-longer-study-finds

On One Meal A Day and Weekend Fasting:

Michael and Maša Ofei, the creators behind The Minimalist Vegan—a website, a blog, a podcast—talk about OMAD: https://theminimalistvegan.com/

Join the OMAD Diet community: https://omaddiet.com/community/

From the Harvard School of Public Health: the straight skinny on whether intermittent fasting helps you lose weight: https://www.hsph.harvard.edu/nutritionsource/healthy-weight/diet-reviews/intermittent-fasting/

More on fasting and weight loss, from: https://www.ncbi.nlm.nih.gov/pubmed/28537332

A link to Well And Good, an excellent wellness site with a good piece on fasting and "brain benefits": https://www.wellandgood.com/good-advice/intermittent-fasting-brain-benefits/

A slightly technical but very comprehensive piece from *Nutrition Journal* on the many studies relating to metabolic changes caused by caloric restriction, from intermittent fasting to OMAD to holiday fasts: https://www.ncbi.nlm.nih.gov/pmc/articles/PMC3200169/?tool=pubmed

A link to The Diet Doctor, a reputable and believable site about newer approaches to eating, like the keto diet, low-carb diets and general, and more: https://www.dietdoctor.com/

Dr. Jason Fung, a Canadian nephrologist and world-leading expert on intermittent fasting and low carb diets (especially for treating people with type 2 diabetes), has written three bestselling health books and co-founded the Intensive Dietary Management program

Alternate Day Fasting is the dietary strategy that has the most research behind it. Much of it was done by Dr. Krista Varady, an assistant professor of nutrition with the University of Illinois—Chicago. She wrote a book about her strategy, *The Every-Other-Day Diet*

The harsh facts on fruit juice as nothing more than a sugary beverage, from the respected medical journal, *The Lancet*: https://www.thelancet.com/journals/landia/article/PIIS2213-8587(14)70013-0/fulltext

On Near-Infrared Radiation (and Placebos)

Read *The Ultimate Guide to Red Light Therapy* by Ari Whitten for more information on Near-Infrared Radiation

An excellent piece on fact vs fiction in light therapy as a benefit to health, from the Illuminative Engineering Society: https://

www.ies.org/fires/the-science-of-near-infrared-lighting-fact-or-fiction/

An abstract on research regarding "open placebos" and back pain: https://www.ncbi.nlm.nih.gov/pmc/articles/PMC5113234/

An article on "open placebos" in treating hay fever: https://journals.plos.org/plosone/article?id=10.1371/journal.pone.0192758

On Vitamins and Mineral Supplements:

A great reference on the vitamins and minerals the body needs and where to get them, from the NHS: https://www.nhs.uk/conditions/vitamins-and-minerals/iron/

A comprehensive study of Sunlight and Vitamin D: https://www.ncbi.nlm.nih.gov/pmc/articles/PMC3897598/

Renowned health expert Jane Brody talks about the ineffectiveness of supplements in her *New York Times* column: https://www.nytimes.com/2016/11/15/well/eat/studies-show-little-benefit-in-supplements.html

A nice fact sheet on Vitamin D from the University of Florida: http://edis.ifas.ufl.edu/pdffiles/FY/FY20700.pdf

On Sleep and Sleep Monitoring:

Why you need a good night's sleep from the National Institute of Health: https://newsinhealth.nih.gov/2013/04/benefits-slumber

The danger of sleep deprivation: https://www.medicalnewstoday.com/articles/307334.php

The CDC tells you how much sleep you need at any age: https://www.cdc.gov/sleep/about_sleep/how_much_sleep.html

A lot of good information from Johns Hopkins' Sleep Disorders Center: https://www.hopkinsmedicine.org/johns_hopkins_bayview/medical_services/specialty_care/sleep_disorders_center/

The cognitive benefits or a good night's sleep: https://www.ncbi.nlm.nih.gov/pubmed/25052368/%EF%BB%BF

The awful impact of a lack of sleep: https://www.ncbi.nlm.nih.gov/pmc/articles/PMC3619301/

How sleep affects athletes' performance: https://www.sleep.org/articles/how-sleep-affects-athletes/

On Journaling:

Psychologist Shilagh Mirgain, PhD, how journaling may lead us to a deeper understanding: https://uwhealth.org/news/the-benefits-of-journaling/48224

An awesome interview on the positive effects of *gratitude* on the human mind, from *Psychology Today*: https://www.psychologytoday.com/us/blog/prefrontal-nudity/201211/the-grateful-brain

A smart little website on journaling that gives some good tips on what to try and how to get started: https://tinybuddha.com/blog/10-journaling-tips-to-help-you-heal-grow-and-thrive/

Read James Pennebaker's groundbreaking book, *Opening It Up By Writing it Down*

The Artist's Way: an essential tool for helping your creativity blossom (including some valuable tips on journaling)

A summary of how writing and speaking—communication skills in general—are linked: https://journals.sagepub.com/doi/abs/10.3102/00346543066001053

ABOUT THE AUTHOR

Brad Munson is an author and editor of fiction and nonfiction. Based in Los Angeles, he has written about health and wellness for decades, including an eight-year stint as editor of *Diabetes Insight*, a monthly audio/print publication for physicians and the members of the treatment team.